Happy Colon, Happy Soul

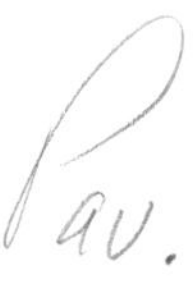

Happy Colon, Happy Soul

An Exploration of Why and How We Share Food

KAREN GIESBRECHT

RESOURCE *Publications* • Eugene, Oregon

HAPPY COLON, HAPPY SOUL
An Exploration of Why and How We Share Food

Resource Publications
An Imprint of Wipf and Stock Publishers
199 W. 8th Ave., Suite 3
Eugene, OR 97401

www.wipfandstock.com

PAPERBACK ISBN: 978-1-5326-8225-4
HARDCOVER ISBN: 978-1-5326-8226-1
EBOOK ISBN: 978-1-5326-8227-8

Manufactured in the U.S.A. 05/16/19

For the friends I get to work with as we share the food we have with our hungry neighbours. And for those who give generously, so we can throw lavish dinner parties. And for those addressing the broken parts of our food system, so some day we will not have so many in our circles who know deep hunger. If I named you all, it would be a very long list.

Contents

Acknowledgements

THANK-YOU TO MY PARENTS, who taught me to cook from scratch, to regularly welcome all sorts of people around our table, and to live out what I believe really matters, and to Clarence, who raised me with the balance of humour and grit needed for this work. Thank-you to everyone I have had the pleasure of sharing a home with since my UBC days, when I started on this journey, especially when dinner was already cooking as I got home from a long day. When you let me debrief the hard stories, I do not even mind if you label the choicest leftovers with "delight" or "surprise" so I will not eat them.

Thank-you to Jonathan for articulating that we can do something about haphazard food charity, and for all the doors you have opened for me these past seven years. Thank-you to all who encouraged me to finish this, especially Karen, Louise, and Lee, and to my parents and Robert for catching my grammatical sins.

Thank-you to all the volunteers who show up faithfully, week after week, to the community dinners across Vancouver, especially those who chop the onions, and those who stay until the last dish is put away and the compost is carried outside. I appreciate all the ways you feed me, and all the times you try my ideas (even when it means a little more work).

Preface

Years ago, while visiting friends in the United Kingdom, we had been lingering over brunch, joking about how I should write a quack diet book one day that would make fun of fad diets and people who fall for their marketing gimmicks. We mused about how I would have to publish it under a pen name, as I had taken an oath as a dietitian to promote only good nutritional science. This was years before gut bacteria were widely understood to provide so many benefits, and before probiotics was a common term, though centuries after many cultures around the world had figured out that, if they fermented certain foods—kimchi, miso soup, kombucha, yogurt and sauerkraut—those who ate them felt better. We decided the book would naturally include some self-help advice, and thus would be named, "Happy Colon, Happy Soul." The title sounds posher in a British accent, so the book would be released in England first.

More recently, a friend took a summer-long gourmet culinary course. For the first half of the course, students were instructed to follow recipes exactly. For the second half of the course, they were not allowed to look at recipes—by then they were learning to cook by heart. While I remain interested in the fads, trends and systems that inspire how people eat, this is not a cookbook. It is an exploration of why and how we share food with others, particularly those who cannot adequately stock their own kitchens. These are thoughts about how to nourish our communities, and our souls, but in more of a spirit-of-the-law, rather than letter-of-the-law kind of way. Take it as a second-half-of-cooking-school recipe, without any quack science, and only occasional self-help references.

This is a work of nonfiction, though I have taken a few creative liberties with details in order to respect the privacy of my friends (and keep them as friends), when I do not remember the exact details, or, occasionally, just for a bit of poetic fun. Most of it is true, though, even the story about the attempt to eradicate all broccoli from planet earth.

Many of these stories do have the real names and places of the amazing individuals who have nourished me, and with whom I get to work as we figure out how to support our neighbors on the margins. We regularly witness the vulnerable places that hunger brings people to, literally and figuratively, and experience the things that erode or build up agency. It takes an extended community of practice to explore how we can best respond. I once heard a pastor refer to how his church did "a feeding of people," which made me cringe for the distant tone he assumed. His sentiment did not synchronize with how I experience my work. I hope that by the time you put this book down, you will be inspired to invest in a different approach to human need.

Introduction

Translating into Food

"You are not acting like Jesus."

How would you react if someone said this to you? You, readers, may know Jesus as Creator, Teacher, Counselor, cartoonish felt board character, baby that we carol about at Christmas, or just two syllables that slip out when you are frustrated. Regardless, we can probably all agree on this: being told that one is un-Jesus-like is not a compliment. Rather, it is a trigger for our bodies to tense up, preparing to defend ourselves.

Now imagine someone did not just *say* it. "You! Are Not! Acting! Like Jesus!" He yelled it so that everyone in the room with you could hear. And that someone was a drunk-beyond-all-rationality man bellowing at the community meal you were overseeing.

I had just told Rolly he would have to leave before dinner was ready. Tension in the church hall had been rising as he grew louder and more unpredictable. Other days I would have let him stay, knowing he would do better with a good meal in him. However, a fight had broken out the week before over perceived racial slurs and everyone was more on edge than usual.

Our regular cook had not shown up that night, opting for either a date with a beer bottle or a paid labor gig he had somehow talked his way into. After some scrambling, the rest of our volunteer cooks were getting a handle on the meal, though we would be serving at least twenty minutes late. We had planned to make breaded chicken and potato salad with cilantro from the garden boxes planted along the south side of the church that hosted the meal. At this program, we liked to make things from scratch, and tried to find ways to engage as many community members as possible. Our menu plan that night included toasting the donated sourdough bread, smashing it into crumbs, seasoning it, and using that to coat the chicken before baking it. An hour before the doors were to open, the chicken was still partially frozen, we had just started boiling the potatoes, and I was wondering why I had not bought chicken nuggets.

I had twisted my ankle a few days before this exchange, and every step was painful. Unfortunately, with my colleague out of town, I could not take the day off. I was well aware that there were several other guests in the room who were also under the influence of some mind-altering substance, but they were behaving as peacefully as the sober guests. I was also conscious of the need for fairness, and I did not want to ask Rolly to leave unnecessarily. Yet, my gut instinct was that there would be problems if he stayed, so I hobbled over to him.

Sometimes, being an introvert gives me an edge. I cannot instantly think of something intelligent to say in heated moments, especially when I am simultaneously reasoning with a drunk person, assessing how a large meal is coming along, trying not to shift weight onto my right foot, planning what to say to a community group that is visiting our program for the first time, and intensely conscious of what the other ninety-nine people in the room are thinking as they watch me. I pondered briefly on how un-Jesus-like I can be, and I had a wave of childlike angst, since I wanted to be seen as a good little Sunday school kid. I also had some vague thought about how I had not been taught to handle situations like this in grade school, Bible school, dietitian's school, or leadership school.

Early the next morning, woken by the pain in my ankle, I thought about how I should have simply told Rolly the truth. "I am trying to be like Jesus, and I know I fall far short. I want to give you food, to ease the hunger pangs you are feeling, stabilize your blood sugar, let you taste some much needed kindness, and make it easier on whomever you meet next, but there are complicating factors. Really, I just want to put my head on your shoulder and cry right now, but I cannot because there are a lot of other hungry people here, including my Most Difficult Volunteer, and I am feeling frustrated at being abandoned by my colleague. If you leave, I think I will be able to cope with everything else. Kyrie eleison."

And then my thoughts rolled into prayer. "Jesus, I am trying to feed you, but you could make it a little easier on me. I can handle when you show up at my community meals disguised as a bristly, smelly, ravenous homeless person, but being shamed in front of all the other Jesus look-alikes is not fair. If we are going to keep on caring for the least of these in Vancouver, you have got to play your part. I will own that I was looking at my cell phone last week, not watching the sidewalk, but you could have sent an angel to wrap his hands around my ankle as I stumbled. When this body is functional, I can act justly and love mercy. I did not need this lesson to walk humbly. Or maybe I did."

But in the moment, I just stared at Rolly as I tried to think of something to say that would make sense to him in his altered state—something that would be kind yet firm, compassionate yet fair, boundaried yet graceful, and maybe even a bit funny to diffuse the tension. It must have taken longer than he was comfortable with, or the Spirit finally decided to intervene, because Rolly spun around and left the building without any more accusations.

Feeding people, and making a space where those on the margins, or any strangers who enter our lives, are welcomed is a delightful and difficult task. There is no manual on how to do this. Someone could try to write one, but no two moments are ever the same, and the way each of us prefers to eat is as unique and personal as our signatures. Still, here, I am going to try, and, hopefully, by articulating what I have learned from my various teachers—my hungry friends, wise professors, faithful volunteers, favorite authors, generous family, trial and error—we can learn to nourish ourselves and our neighbors a little better.

The recipe for sharing food with one's community could be as simple as a generous cup of love + variety + good boundaries. Translating that into food takes more adaptability, creativity and community-mindedness than any one person or organization has on its own. This book is the story of the collaboration I get to witness in the church basements and community halls across my city.

Church Cookies

In feeding others, I am also trying to find my place in church. I am doing what I can to build up the beautiful, messy, inspiring, difficult, worthy conglomeration of compassion and hospitality that this world and I still need. Sara Miles, in *Take this Bread*,[1] refers to her earlier understanding of church as a Jesus-and-cookies experience. At a church my brother used to be part of, a huggable older lady known as Cookie Jan would stand outside the sanctuary on Sunday mornings, greeting people with treats. One morning when I was visiting, the service had started and I was standing near the back of the sanctuary with my brother as he held his two-year-old daughter. Neither was singing, but they were engaging with the music when their friend Eddie wandered in. Eddie has a good heart, but he wears the scars of a difficult life. He is not the kind of guy a protective dad would normally hand his daughter over to, nor would a toddler normally allow herself to be taken from her daddy's arms by someone like him. But Eddie came over, whispered something about cookies, and then lifted Elli and walked out of the room. They were back a minute later, Elli pleased with herself for being allowed to double fist her snack, and Eddie pleased for having done something nice for his friends.

1. Miles, *Take This Bread*, v.

That moment struck me as symbolic of all that is beautiful about church and food—what else brings trust and connection between such unlikely friends? But, there were some things wrong with the scene. Cookie Jan had cheap, white-sugar-white-flour-fiberless treats. I resisted the temptation to read the labels on her packages, but I am pretty sure there was modified canola, soybean, palm and/or sunflower oil in them, and neither the ingredients nor the packaging could claim anything about sustainability. The plastic wrap was going to end up in the landfill, and the soil where the wheat, sugar and other ingredients were grown was probably not restored with compost or integrated pest management practices. Those who ate the cookies that morning also sang about loving God and neighbor, yet were mostly oblivious to the lives and working conditions of the people who grew the base ingredients of their snack. I enjoyed one of Jan's cookies that morning, too, but it did not sit right with me.

Church Basements

I stumbled into the niche of community dinners served in church basements, and have found no parallel that is so welcoming, faithful, delightful, eclectic, and caring—both for me, and for everyone else who walks through the doors week after week. What started out as an occasional volunteer experience—partly looking for an excuse to take a break from my textbooks, partly looking for something to make my university student life feel less like a game—has turned into a vocation.

Coordinating such programs is not what I imagined I would do when I filled out applications for a degree in dietetics, but since so much good work related to poverty reduction, food security, social support, reconciliation and overall well-being is currently done in church basements, shelters, missions and faith-based food programs, this is where I will stay for now. Bloom where you are planted.

For a report at an annual general meeting of the church where I was accused of not acting like Jesus, I calculated one year that I got to manage more than two hundred hours of volunteer time each week to serve about 250 plates of food. We could have served those meals with less labor, but that is not the point. The food is not our end goal, but rather it is the context where the alchemy (or the ministry, to use the more contextual vernacular) happens.

The Setting Matters

Sharing food with my vulnerable neighbors takes me to diverse care settings all over Vancouver. I went to see Lee, a friend, of sorts, in the hospital one day. She was temporarily committed to the Psychiatric Assessment Unit, against her will, but her being there was a relief. Lee's ability to care for herself while out on the streets was declining at an alarming rate, but she did not seem to grasp how dire her life was. Although autonomy must be highly valued, there are times when care should be forced on people. I do not envy those who are in a position to make that decision, but I do pray for them.

I have known Lee for at least ten years, and she had not had a home for nine and a half of those years, not counting the stints she claimed to be living with an extravagantly rich boyfriend. Lee had attached herself to the church I attended years ago, and managed to get invited out for lunch most weeks. When she joined the group I was eating with, she would seem oblivious to the chatter going on around her, then occasionally make comments that showed she was following our conversations closely, and she had often read the book, seen the movie, or met the person we were discussing.

During my visit, Lee and I chatted about the medications she did not like, the people she did not like (which was most of the staff and other patients, except the dominatrix who allegedly charged $200 per hour for her services), the likelihood that all of her doctors were crack addicts, and the romantic thriller she was reading.

Lee also told me that she was hungry. A long season of undernourishment, plus altered metabolism from the anti-psych medications she was given, was taking a toll. When dinner arrived, we walked out of her room and found a seat at one of the tables in the ward's common room. It was one of the saddest scenes I could imagine. There were about a dozen people, all at their lowest, some there voluntarily, many not, most on heavy medications that their body was struggling to adjust to, and a meal of sweet and sour pork with carrots, rice, steamed carrots, and carrot cake in rectangular plastic bowls on old rectangular trays, with tea made from water that smelled like coffee.

Having worked on that menu in my early years as a dietitian, I knew something was wrong with what showed up on her tray. No one would plan an entrée, side dish and dessert with the same base ingredient. The psych ward was the last to be served at that facility, so some parts of the planned meal must have run out while the first nine hundred trays were served, with leftovers from a previous meal substituted in.

The way the patients were eating was even more distressing. Most people were sitting alone, eating with plastic forks. One man even had his tray perched on the little ledge by the payphone in the corner of the room. Only one patient was engaging with another, tenderly helping him navigate the food in front of him. When Lee saw me looking at the pair, she loudly whispered that the woman helping was the one who could earn $200 an hour.

The staff on shift were at the nurses' station, not paying attention to how patients were eating. It was mid-evening, and I believe they care, and hopefully they are more present during the day. The entire scene renewed my commitment to feed people well. The setting—physical and relational—matters as much as the food on the plate.

Shifts in Understanding

Father Greg Boyle,[2] a Jesuit priest who spent much of his life working with gang members in Los Angeles, talks about how our goal should not be service to the vulnerable, but kinship. I cannot claim to feel a family loyalty with all my colorful volunteers and program

2. Boyle, *Tattoos on the Heart.*

participants, but it comes close with a good number of my crew. Seeing people as my kin, rather than as poor souls who need my help, feels like a significant shift in posturing, and thus a shift in my energy and in how much of my heart I invest.

With a foot in both the church and charity worlds, I have perceived a shift in understanding within many programs from assuming we know what needs to be done and asking (praying) for support in that, to looking for what signs of hope exist in a neighborhood, and breathing life into those—an asset-based community development approach. I have seen a shift from a focus on relief work (though there is time for that) to prioritizing development, which is harder and slower, but ultimately more rewarding. There has been a shift in seeing food programs as valuable for reducing hunger to seeing them as valuable for the social capital they provide. Free food treats the symptoms of poverty, but only adequate income will ultimately address hunger. Supportive programs have shifted from focusing on rules and boundaries to prioritizing trauma-informed care. We have shifted toward seeing people as more than physical bodies healed by science and nutrients, counting emotions and our relationship with food as legitimate indicators of health. There has been a renewed interest in cooking and traditional food preservation techniques, as we went too far down the processed and convenience aisles. And with food itself, we have shifted from focusing on fat as the deep source of most of our health problems to understanding that it is sugar.

All these shifts take a lot of listening, reading, reflecting, vegetable chopping, pot scrubbing, and going back, again-and-again, into the kitchens, the dining rooms, the lives of our relations. By wandering through Vancouver's food programs, we will engage in a little theopoetics, following Mary Oliver's poem, "Sometimes."[3]

> Instructions for living a life:
> Pay attention.
> Be astonished.
> Tell about it.

3. Oliver, *Red Bird*, 37.

Chapter 1

Sharing Food

My Historic Commitment

CHARITABLE FOOD PROGRAMS HAVE turned into a career for me, but maybe also a calling (on my good days). I aspire to live up to what David Brooks articulates in *The Road to Character*:

> A person who embraces a calling does not take a direct route to self-fulfillment. She is willing to surrender the things that are most dear, and by seeking to forget herself and submerge herself, she finds a purpose that defines and fulfills her. Such vocations almost always involve tasks that transcend a lifetime. They almost always involve throwing yourself into a historical process. They involve compensating for the brevity of life by finding membership in a historic commitment.[1]

The historic commitment I landed in is hunger. Really, it is the problem of poverty and injustice, not a lack of food or cookbooks. I must admit, though, that I did not get into this field because I understood or believed I could contribute to any complex, global historical process. I just needed a summer job.

1. Brooks, *The Road to Character*, 46.

At the end of my first year as a University of British Columbia dietetics student, I applied for any job that would allow me to stay in Vancouver and provide a sufficient income to pay my expenses through the next school year. Around the same time that I met Lee, I started volunteering at a church-run weekly community meal because of Dan, a charming friend-of-a-friend, who told me that a weekly church dinner needed female volunteers to help make the few women who attended feel more at ease amongst the gruff male majority.

A few weeks of volunteering at that church dinner landed me a summer job in a food recovery program in Vancouver's roughest—and one of Canada's poorest—neighborhoods. At the time, I knew little about hunger or other poverty-related challenges, but as my colleagues and I worked our way through cases of donated, partially melted and refrozen Häagen-Dazs Cappuccino Gelato, I began to develop what is turning into a lifelong pilgrimage focused on just, sustainable and nourishing food for our more vulnerable neighbors.

I remember feeling bewildered at our freezer full of ice cream which was perfectly safe to eat, but unacceptable to sell, and inappropriate for many of the organization's programs at the time. Eating that ice cream, given my limited student budget, felt indulgent, and wrong on several levels.

Now, years later, I better understand the systems in place that led me to the basement of an old church, with so much good food around me, and people just outside our office doors who were struggling to survive. Looking back, I can see how my membership in this historic commitment began, but my start really came from a crush on a guy called Dan, and then from an abundance of coffee-flavored gelato.

Long Slow Heart-Shifts

I once heard my wise, grown-up friend Karen talk about the long, slow heart-shift that we experience as we move through life. She was giving a talk about learning to offer hospitality, and I have been paying attention ever since to how my heart and approach to the world have shifted in the past decade. I am also more conscious of when my heart shifts quickly, within a few hours, from hope to despair.

I went out one February night with a mobile outreach van and two mission outreach workers. A few nights a week, they fill the van with sandwiches, hot chocolate, socks, blankets, and other basic necessities, then start on their route. For the next few hours, until the sandwiches are all given out, they drive down the back alleys of Vancouver, looking for the people that many others try not to see.

Ricky, the driver, had moved to Vancouver from South America years ago, and seemed to have the perfect mix of patience, compassion, humor, faith, and wisdom for his job. Andrew's role was to fill the snack bags, navigate, keep stats, organize the back shelves, and jump out of the van whenever we saw someone in a place where we could not easily pull over. He also got to operate the remote control for the light mounted on top of the van to do a quick sweep of parks when they knew someone was likely hidden there.

"Hey, man," Ricky would say as he idled the van next to someone in an alley, "how ya doin' tonight? You want some hot chocolate?" His accent made him unintimidating as he leaned out his window, enunciating all three of *chocolate's* syllables. Two of the guys we found declined the hot chocolate, almost apologetically, since they were already nursing a beer. I had not thought about it before, but I guess the two flavors do not pair particularly well. Most accepted it gladly. A few also asked for a warm layer of clothing.

It was a cold night, near freezing. We found someone with no shoes wandering in an alley between a Baptist church and a YMCA. My feet were cold, and I had two pairs of socks, plus boots, plus a seat in a heated van. Jean was 60, coming down off speed, which he had not been using for long, was planning on sleeping on his brother's couch that night, preferred high-arch shoes, and was originally from Quebec. We learned all that in the first eleven seconds or so. He was wearing a thin jacket, so we invited him to sit down in the van, and helped him put on dry socks and a pair of shoes more stylish than supportive, but that was all we had with us in his size. Andrew gave Jean a pair of gloves and a sweater, which he tried to put on in that order. We eventually got the gloves and his jacket off him, the sweater on, then his jacket, and then the gloves, again. Andrew had to help him out of the van, and ensured that Jean had the mission's contact information for when he was ready for a change.

I saw a different side of Vancouver that night than I usually see. I had no idea there was a camper van village behind an industrial park in the middle of the city, but I now know which alleys have the most cast-off furniture, and where I would "camp" if I ever found myself needing to.

The first few hours of the evening were hard to describe—fun is not the right word, but it captures an element of it. We laughed as I started to roll my window down, ready to greet someone leaning into a bin, then realizing it was an apartment tenant throwing out his recycling, not someone looking for a bit of recoupable value. One guy who did appear to be homeless accepted the sandwich I offered, and by way of thanks, said with a thick Scottish accent, "Things could be worse. I could be feeling this bad *and* be English."

It was touching to see people on the street express care for someone they knew who was nearby, giving us directions to find their buddies and explaining what help they might need. It felt good to be so welcomed and appreciated by those we met. Most of them, at least. Many blessed us as we were about to drive on.

But as the evening wore on, my feet got colder, my blood sugar dipped, and I got tired, it got harder. I wanted to get home and crawl into my warm bed, but was conscience-stricken, since none of the men, nor the two women we found, would be doing that. The compassion I felt at the start of the evening turned to sad desperation and helpless annoyance—both at these peoples' unwillingness to accept a ride back to the shelter, and the system that made that an unappealing choice.

Where the Heart-Shift is Needed

I am increasingly uncomfortable with long food lineups. There are better ways to meet nutrient needs for those who cannot afford food, shelter and other necessities. Food lines are not dignifying, nor easy, for guests, staff or volunteers. The last time I helped out with one, we fed 437 people in just over an hour. I had the role of handing full trays to the guests as they shuffled past the serving line. It was a Friday, and the organization had a patron who donated fish on Fridays. It is challenging to cook fish for large crowds, but cream sauce helps. Potato salad and cauliflower had also been donated that week, so they rounded out the meal.

The price of cauliflower had come up several times in recent conversations, one friend saying she had spent $12 on a head of it for a Christmas dinner. The spike in price at grocery stores had led to an overabundance somewhere in the supply chain, so several cases of edible, if slightly browning, cauliflower had been donated to the organization hosting this meal.

In any course on serving food, students will be taught that presentation matters. Consider colors and texture as much as flavors, nutrition, and what you can manage in your kitchen space. Avoid, at all costs, the discreditable monochromatic meal of white fish with a cream sauce, potatoes and steamed cauliflower. Although the food looked tasty, and I had long since passed any requisite foodservice courses, I struggled to shake a niggling concern over getting marks docked for this particular meal.

Of the 437 people to whom I handed the tray, which at least was brightened up by a perfectly ripe yellow banana (a rarity in the charity food world), fewer than half of the people made eye contact with me. Only about ten percent engaged me in a brief conversation. Another ten percent made no acknowledgment of me. They took the tray as they shuffled by with their eyes averted. The rest bobbed their head and said "thank you" quietly, so I mostly just heard ". . . you . . . you . . . you . . . " as the individuals got their meals. There was one child in this crowd and about forty older women, many who were around the same age as my mom, triggering another level of empathy in me.

While handing out the trays, resisting the urge to hug a few of the people walking past me, or go sit with those who were not talking to the people eating beside them, or stopping the whole line so I could call the organization's executive director and convince her there is a better way to share food, I was chatting with the volunteer beside me. Blake had recently been released from jail, and was trying to get his life on track. He had been given kitchen duty for much of his time inside, which he had liked, since it gave him access to good food and a chance to perfect his pasta sauce recipe. His secret was to start by *slowly* caramelizing the onions with a bit of brown sugar.

Since leaving jail, Blake had visited a number of free food programs and had put on more weight than he was comfortable with. He had taken to skipping breakfast to cut down on calories, so between focusing on our guests, not dropping any trays, ignoring the ache in my arm that started around tray #283, and planning what I was going to say to the executive director, I tried to help Blake understand why eating in the morning matters, and what effect skipping breakfast could have on the decisions he would make through the rest of the day, especially on his food choices. I hoped it was a useful conversation, though we could have been more focused if it had taken place in a better setting. I intend not to retire before this particular food line has been transformed, even though it is hosted by one of the larger, more established organizations in Vancouver, and is a significant asset in the continuum of support for our most vulnerable neighbors.

Wayne's Heart-Shift

"Hey, are you the one who's responsible for all the changes?" Wayne asked me one day at a smaller community lunch, his tone inferring he was not happy with the new service style the volunteer team was trying. I had been invited to spend some time with the church food program, helping the church align it with the kind of justice that was preached on Sundays. I had avoided sitting near Wayne during my previous visits, as he seemed quick to disapprove of whatever and whoever displeased him that day. Wayne's accusation came one hour before he would give me a hug as he left the church hall.

Wayne had settled into the back alley just outside the church, and was on a first-name basis with almost everyone who passed through its doors. He would make himself quite at home whenever food was served at a service or mid-week program. It had been a rough winter, though, and he frequently came to the weekly community lunch with little appetite, knocked down by an array of bugs and viruses.

Wayne, having lost his teeth somewhere along his journey, is a petite man with the thinnest chin I have ever seen, but people still moved when he hovered over them, informing any newcomers they had mistakenly chosen *his* seat. A few weeks earlier, I had been in a conversation with someone else at Wayne's table, when he had joined in. I had learned that Wayne and his clan hold their women in high esteem. The only thing they value more is their freedom. Having spent almost the entire decade of the 1990s in the Nebraska State Pen, Wayne especially valued his freedom. To him, it seemed to be a rational choice to make his home in the shadow of a downtown church.

Wayne's story is allegedly written down and locked away in a friend's safety deposit box, with instruction to be released only after he dies. It is a good story, he assured me, but it would implicate some powerful people in Vancouver who would not allow him to live if certain details became public. Wayne had flown to Florida several times, picked up a nondescript car with a few bricks of cocaine in the trunk, and leisurely driven back to Vancouver. He would sell his stash and make enough to live very comfortably for a year until he went again. Regrettably, on one trip, something had tipped someone off, and he thus ended up in jail, walking out alive only because his clients had made it known that he was an important figure. Wayne has the gift of storytelling, and whether or not the details were true, I developed a bit of admiration for him after hearing his tale.

And thus I felt mildly affronted when he told me that neither he, nor the rest of the guests in the room, liked what the volunteers were trying. Up until a few weeks before this conversation, guests at this lunch had lined up outside the church and, at precisely 11:30, filed into the church hall, past a table where a volunteer had written out a list of sandwiches on a whiteboard which corresponded to the rows of lovingly made, plastic-wrapped, frozen, defrosted sandwiches on the table behind where they stood. Each guest would read the whiteboard and tell the volunteer what kind of sandwich he or she wanted. The volunteer would dutifully hand over the right sandwich, and cross it off the board when that particular flavor was gone. The guests would then shuffle down the table, point to the two cookies they favored, and another volunteer would hand them their dessert choice in a napkin.

The system had been honed to a smooth, quick process after a decade or so, and everyone—guests and volunteers—knew what to expect. More importantly (to some), a few of the regulars knew how to work the system, get to the front of the line, and be at a table and biting into their sandwich within seconds of the doors opening. Now, the volunteers were trying out table-service, though it was taking a few weeks to orchestrate everyone into a cohesive rhythm.

"Yeah, nobody likes this," Wayne went on. "I sometimes have to wait for my sandwich. If I line up first, I should be served first." Fair point. But Wayne was missing something. Most of the volunteers understood the changes by then, although a few were still muttering don't-fix-what-ain't-broke type phrases. Lining up, as the guests were expected to do, with volunteers clearly holding a more privileged role on the other side of the table, is belittling. The team had created a lovely setting in all other ways—someone was playing the piano that was set in the corner of the hall, the tablecloths were colorful, water jugs were on the table, baristas came around with coffee, and there was some of the most beautiful textile art I have ever seen on the walls.

Without preaching (I hoped), I tried to help Wayne see that it was okay to wait a few minutes. He would certainly still get something to eat. I also tried to help Wayne understand that it would be fair if someone who was less aggressive than those who elbowed their way through the doors first was served before he was. Wayne conceded that maybe I had a fair line of reasoning, and I left the conversation at that.

A few minutes later, I was chatting with the volunteer who was ladling up the soup. I had done that task the week before, and I knew one's arm got tired after the first few dozen bowls. Dora, a lovely, if somewhat timid volunteer, came and quietly asked me if Wayne could have another bowl of soup. Wayne was not feeling well that day. I had seen him blanch a little when the sandwich was offered to him. He had likely eaten something earlier that had sat in his pocket for too long. I had no more authority to allow it than Dora did, but she perceived that I did, or perceived that it would be better if I got in trouble for making the wrong call.

It was the practice in this program never to give out a second bowl of soup, but we were near the end of the lunch service, and so I quietly carried one over to Wayne's table and set it in front of him, neither interrupting the story he was telling his neighbors, nor drawing attention lest the rule-following volunteers notice I was breaking tradition. It is important to treat everyone equally, but sometimes a subversive second bowl of soup can communicate that change is okay, and that there will be enough, even if the first people through the door are not the first ones with food in front of them.

I was not even sure Wayne had noticed that I had put the soup in front of him until I got the shy hug as he passed me on his way out. Reflecting back now, I am trying to imagine why he preferred the lineup to being served at a table. Is that what institutionalization does to someone? Does he not believe he deserves better service? Is he only able to look out for himself?

A few of the long-time volunteers who were used to their routines took the sentiments that Wayne and his ilk expressed as proof that the changes we were trying were a failure, and we should return to the old serving style. I tried to remain open to that, though it had felt so wrong when I was assigned the role of cookie lady, doling out each person's allotment (maybe an extra half if there was a broken piece, for those bold enough to ask). The only redeeming part of my role that day was learning that the men living rough in Vancouver's downtown peninsula seem to have a two-to-one preference for peanut butter cookies over chocolate chip. For anyone who plans dessert for programs in that neighborhood, let this important tidbit help you bake accordingly.

Eight months later, when I visited this same program, now a sit-down dinner with table service and more variety in the menu, Wayne found me and told me that the setting was better than he expected. This was more validation for me to keep going than any raise or new contract I have ever received.

The Cost of Being Poor

We know so much about wellness and resilience, and have enough food—so much that we fill dumpsters with groceries that are still edible—and yet so many struggle. "Hunger amid plenty remains one of the inexcusable conundrums of our time," Peter Ladner wrote in *The Urban Food Revolution*.[2] If you have read this far, I imagine you have had experience with individuals on the margins, or at least donated to a program that addresses hunger. I trust you are feeling some draw towards understanding why we need to shift some of the ways we share food. If you are not already convinced, let me introduce you to a few more of my dinner companions.

"Karen, I kinda don't have any underwear. You got any?" Brady asked when he showed up to volunteer for a program I was running. I had known Brady in my university years, and where my life has become increasingly grounded and interesting, his had derailed, and now he was couch-surfing, living without much income, and asking for basic necessities. I had considered Brady

2. Ladner, *The Urban Revolution: Changing the Way We Feed Cities*, 214.

a friend years earlier, and now I was in this awkward position of power over him.

I had lost touch with Brady, so when he had shown up at the dinner one night, not knowing that I was running it, our reunion was bittersweet—glad to see each other, but I sensed he was ashamed of how far his life had slipped into chaos, and he was desperate for support. After he ate, I put him to work "earning" his meal by bussing tables. It restored a bit of balance in our friendship, until he showed up several weeks later and had to admit he was going commando.

Curiously, as I was having breakfast with friends the week before, sitting around a large table with an ocean view, enjoying fresh eggs from their farm and savoring my second cup of coffee, I had received a text from a former colleague saying she had several packages of men's underwear, and would drop them by if I could use them. I responded that I could, figuring I would have a conversation sometime in the near future like the one I was having with Brady. Although it is a stretch to find a scientific correlation between clean skivvies and nutritional status, there must be one, since I have a few stories like this.

Even more curiously, Brady had a large cup of coffee from a neighborhood café in his hand as he presented his request to me. It is possible that someone bought it for him, or that he fished the cup out of the garbage, rinsed it out (hopefully!), and filled it with free coffee from another charity. But it is more likely that he spent the few dollars he had on the coffee, buying legitimacy, even though that forced us to have this delicate conversation, and the feeling of validity would last only as long as the caffeine buzz.

Reflecting out loud with another volunteer later, I wrestled with how to respond in moments like that. It does not feel right to give our limited supplies to someone who chooses to spend what he has on something that I do not even afford myself very often, especially if this would mean that I would have nothing to offer the next guy who asked, someone who had gone even longer without clean base layers. At the same time, I know Brady was really seeking something deeper and more life-giving than underwear.

"I was really poor a while ago," said the other volunteer. "I would do that a lot. Being poor is expensive."

Pictures of Privilege

Being close to people who struggle with so many different manifestations of poverty keeps me conscious of just how unequal the world is, and how privileged I am. Before Lee ended up in the psych ward, while she still held title for being one of the most challenging and charming women on Vancouver's streets, the police dropped her off at my community dinner one night. We ran a shelter one night per week at the time and, uncharacteristically, Lee stayed overnight. She also slept through much of the next day on the couch as we served lunch and cleaned up around her.

At the end of the day, in a rush to get home to dinner with the friends I was sharing my home with, I got Lee and her walker into my car, and asked her where she wanted to go. She did not have an answer. She would not go to one of the local shelters or drop-in centers set up for folks in her position, nor was she keen on her usual places—a library or 24-hour doughnut shop.

Lee was upset that I was not taking her to a movie, as I had suggested I would several weeks earlier—partially wanting to do something fun with her, and partially hoping I could entice her back to my program and connect her with a mental health outreach worker. I had reserved time for her the previous week, but she had not come then.

We drove off the church parking lot, and I headed toward one of the local libraries, still open to suggestions on where Lee would rather go, but receiving none. Finally, she burst out, "I just want to live in a million dollar house!"

I started to say, "Lee, no one gets to live in a million dollar house," but then realized that I do. Casa Blanca, the 103-year-old, four-story house I was renting with several others would probably sell for more than three million. Moments like this make me simultaneously grateful for the privileges I experience, and almost paralyzingly dispirited over the unfairness of life.

"That's a nice car you got. Waddit cost?" a voice stopped me another day when I was running late to a meeting. I was a little over-caffeinated from the first two meetings of the day. I had a lot to do before the end of the day, and I did not have time for this lady's accusations. It did not feel kind, but I tried to brush her off.

The lady was not deterred. "Must be expensive. What did it cost?" She had a walker, a few scraggly facial hairs, an oversized lime-green t-shirt, an edge in her voice, and plenty more marks of a challenging life.

I do not know how to answer questions like this. The car, purchased by my parents with an unexpected inheritance, was brand new a year ago, and nicer than I would have picked, but it does make life easier. I appreciate the heated seats more than I am willing to admit. The back seat held a few days worth of breakfast dishes and the trunk was full of donated groceries that I had to drop off at a food program.

I am often struck by my privilege. I grew up in a solid family, well fed, well educated, well loved. I got to travel, take music lessons, live with some excellent models of hospitality, and be generous with what we had. I can slip into a little self-pity, thinking that I do not own a house, have the salary some of my peers make, or have benefits that will cover the eyeglasses that I will need before too long. And then I have interactions with a woman like this.

"Karen, take time for her," the Spirit nudged, almost audibly. "Our role is to humanize this place," I imagined my friend Tamar would say. It was a line we heard on the radio one day, and we often remind each other of its wisdom.

"This car was an inheritance from my aunt who passed away last year," I said to the woman, which was almost true. It was my great-aunt who had passed away. Aunt Ruth had worked for the City of Vancouver for most of her life, and had saved much of the salary she had made. I also inherited a box of silver cutlery from her: an eight-piece set of forks, knives, soup spoons and dessert spoons, all inscribed with the letter "R." Each piece had arrived in the mail, after she had finished a box of Corn Flakes and sent in a part of the box label. She must have had Corn Flakes for breakfast every morning for years. The silverware is my reminder of what a little thrifty determination can get.

"Oh. I'm so sorry," said the lady with a completely different tone, putting an empathetic hand on my arm. "Hey, what do you get if a porcupine and a snake *get it on*?" she asked, moving her hands to help me visualize the complicated mating ritual.

I realized she was making a joke to cheer me up after my sad revelation. "I don't know," I said, still trying to rush this interaction a little, but I was intrigued with her now. The moment also felt complicated because I was holding my wallet, fishing for coins for the parking meter, unsure of what would be kind and fair. I do not generally give out change, but people whose bodies are craving food or other substances do not necessarily understand my reasoning for that.

"Think!" the lady commanded me, inferring that I was not taking her seriously enough, and also indicating that she wanted my attention, not my money. We made eye contact, and she smiled, saying, "You get barbed wire." She giggled, and that made me laugh, too.

"Have a nice day," I said, and turned to go.

"You, too," she replied as she gripped the handles of her walker. I made it to my meeting on time enough, encouraged by the human interaction, hoping she was as well.

We are formed by what we love, not necessarily by what we are taught in school, or what titles we hold, or what kind of car we drive. This morning, still in my pj's, watching the rain outside, I feel a bit of affection for that woman. I wish I had asked her name.

Sometimes, walking past lineups of mostly men outside the bigger charities in Vancouver, I can see the beauty of each life. And then I think how that vision must have come from some Higher Power. On my own, I see smelly, frustrating people whom I have to manage, not peers I relate to. I pray that God will help me see people with his eyes, and then sometimes get surprised when He does.

People do continually amaze me. I see so many tattered, gruff guys, and can start to believe this is normal, that they are choosing to be in the lineups for free meals, and can think that my occasional presence makes a real difference. I know that is neither a true nor helpful way of looking at the reality in Vancouver, and I feel discouraged when I hear others express such opinions.

Fortunately, I get plenty of reminders that everyone is beloved, full of personality, and worthy of good things. Once in a while, I overhear a conversation like this: ". . . I like their steak, but not their lobster." The voice came from behind me at a shelter meal. A second man responded, "Yeah, they overcook their lobster, and I just don't find it that fresh." The first voice said, "It's hard to find good lobster here." A third voice said, "There is the Sandbar. And that place in Horseshoe Bay." What happened to bring these three men from being lobster connoisseurs to a free dinner? I did not have the chance to ask, but it would have been an interesting story.

Froot Loops in Chocolate Milk

One fall day, on my way home from work at an addictions treatment center, I saw a man standing outside another mission. I did not recognize him, but did recognize the signs of a hard life—tattered clothes, underweight, in need of a haircut and a good scrub. I was a few steps past him when I realized that I had just seen something that will inspire the rest of my working life.

In the previous few hours, I had learned that Brady had been taken into custody. His life had continued to go in the wrong direction, so, for him, jail was probably the best place for a while. Hopefully, he would receive the care, boundaries and clean underwear he needed there. I had also heard from a couple who volunteered in one of my programs, saying they were both in hospital with an inexplicable virus. I offered to stop in and see them on my way home from work. They were in different parts of the hospital and would need someone to move their car before the day was over. Walking toward my car, which I had parked a few blocks away, I ran into another occasional volunteer in one of my programs, and as we chatted, I learned he was not doing well. He was on medical leave from work and was in need of a supportive circle around him. I encouraged him to come join our next community meal. He brightened at the invitation, but that seemed feeble in the shadow of the darkness he was shouldering.

Feeling inadequate, tired, and a little hungry, and yet grateful to be connected to so many in this city, I walked on down East Hastings Street, and saw the man on the street. It was around 5:00 pm, raining a little (this is Vancouver), and daylight was starting to fade.

Earlier that afternoon, I had spent an hour with clients in early stages of drug detox talking about why eating regularly matters, and how to address their food cravings, especially for sugar. We had talked about the difference between microwaving a cheap can of ravioli, and preparing a meal as our grandparents would have done—taking several hours to gather ingredients from the garden or neighborhood market and cooking from scratch. Not only would that homemade food have tasted better and been far more nourishing, but the conversation that would have happened as the family cooked together could have helped address the kind of factors that had driven the guys into their out-of-control addictions. I hoped my clients had begun to believe that investing a little more time in preparing their meals could generate considerable Return-On-Investment.

In that conversation, we also somehow got on to the subject of "rabbit starvation," or protein poisoning, a phenomenon that happens when hunters or foragers eat primarily lean game meat. In winter months, they may get enough calories and protein, but not enough fat, and thus their bodies begin to starve. Without enough fat in the foods we eat, we cannot absorb certain nutrients, and some fats are essential building blocks for new cells.

So, with all this in my thoughts, I walked past a man, a deserving human, my neighbor—in the good Samaritan way of seeing people—standing outside on a street corner, alone, in the rain, at dinner time, eating a big bowl of Froot Loops in chocolate milk.

As I walked the next few blocks, I became conscious of everything that was wrong with that image. I imagined what it would feel like to deaden the hunger in his belly (and brain) with something sweet and fiberless doused with something even sweeter and equally fiberless.

I am not entirely opposed to chocolate milk. It does have some good nutrients, and can be a fair snack when consumed in reasonable amounts, but not alongside other ultra-processed foods. I would even munch on a few Froot Loops occasionally, as there is still some childhood allure around them. Whenever the vitamins versus real food topic comes up in my nutrition talks, or a question about which food really is best, dietitians like to bring up the idea that differently colored foods tend to have different nutrients in them, and so the more colors we eat, the more likely it is that we are getting all the building blocks that our bodies need. But the rule does not hold universally true—Froot Loops do not count. They can lead to a different kind of rabbit starvation.

In a just and fair world, that man would have been debriefing his day with people who knew and cared about him as he arranged plates and cutlery on a table, assembled a salad, ladled stew into a serving bowl, sliced up a fresh loaf of bread, and called his people to the table. He would have been inside, warm and dry. He would have paused before taking his first bite, acknowledging his gratitude for everyone who had a hand in growing and preparing the food he was about to consume. He would have eaten until he was satiated, and then had energy to do a project around his home, or go out for some evening entertainment.

We will return to the ideas of how we share food and the settings that radical hospitality can take us into, but first, let us explore what we eat, or probably *ought* to eat.

Chapter 2

What to Eat

My Clinical Assessment

If I got to be your dietitian, and we met in a clinical setting, I would clear my desk, pull out a copy of my Nutrition Care Plan, and introduce myself. I would ask how your day was going, where you where you were from, and something about your tattoos. If you were one of my clients, you would more than likely be tatted up. Talking about body ink is the quickest way I have found to assess how open someone will be, and thus how to ask my next series of questions. Few things are as equally personal and public, with some thought or story behind each picture. I used to ask people what their first tattoo was, but that often led clients to lift their shirt and expose a little more skin than was necessary for a nutrition assessment.

I would then ask your height, weight, and what your usual weight was, or what feels like a healthy weight to you. I ask this because weight is also relatively easy to talk about, although the topic can quickly get more personal. If you seemed concerned (or obsessed, preoccupied, or plagued) about your weight, I would make the point that it is just one measure of health, and although the easiest to measure, it is wiser to focus on healthy rhythms, and not try to change your weight, especially in early stages of recovery from addiction, trauma, illness, or some other life-derailing chaos.

The assessment would follow up with a few more medical questions about diabetes, Hep C, HIV, high blood pressure or heart disease, any allergies or foods you avoid, if you experienced reflux or heartburn, how you were were sleeping, and if you smoked cigarettes. I would ask if you were taking medications or supplements, then about your appetite, fluid intake, and the state of your dental health. If you had questions, or if your answers to my questions concerned me, we would explore an area further.

One client, who had slowly opened up as I asked my questions, wrapped up our conversation by telling me, "I'm a misanthropist. I prefer animals, but you seem alright." I guessed the term's meaning from the context, but I looked it up, and learned that a misanthropist is a person who dislikes all humankind. There is some truth to the adage about the quickest way to a man's heart.

My Less Clinical Assessment

If I got to be your dietitian, and we met in a less clinical setting, and I had to assess the state of your nutritional health, but I could only ask one question, it would be, "*What vegetables have you eaten in the past few days?*" Assuming you are able to get enough to eat, and that you have the freedom to make choices about what to consume—which is not true for many, especially those without an adequate income—you probably choose a reasonably good balance of proteins, fats, and carbohydrates, easing hunger pangs and satisfying your appetite for saltiness, sweetness, crunch and flavor. Vegetables tend to be one of the more time-consuming, perishable parts of our diets, and can be more expensive than packaged convenience foods.

It is all too easy to get out of the habit of purchasing fresh food, leading us to lose our taste for it. But, if prepared with care, vegetables delight us with their variety of colors, textures, tastes and nutrients, and inspire our gut bacterial in-laws to not just live, but to thrive.

"I don't eat vegetables. I was just inside for eight years," someone told me once. I must have looked confused as I worked out the logical connection between leaving prison and no longer eating produce. I thought through conversations with other ex-cons I had met over the years, trying to remember if vegetables had just never come up, or if there was a unique crime for which veg-only diets were an accepted form of punishment.

Without vegetables, it would be challenging to pull together a nutritionally complete diet. Still, even when we know the importance of whole, fresh food, and have it prepared for us, it can be hard to choose to eat vegetables if we have not developed a taste for them. On an annual survey of food of food served at a treatment center, I included the question, "How does the food here impact your recovery?" Given that vegetable consumption is a good proxy measure for overall diet quality and I was curious about the choices the clients made, the next question on the survey was, "What vegetables have you eaten in the past 24 hours?"

One client responded to the first question, "Food is very important to my health, well being and recovery." And to the second question about vegetables, the individual simply wrote, "None." Distressingly, it is a sentiment I hear a little too often.

During a group session at another facility, where we were discussing how food and eating habits are important for health, a client asked, "Shouldn't we tackle our addictions before our diet?" I reviewed how holistic health has to include what we put into our bodies, and how what we eat can impact how we act. Another client, demonstrating active listening skills, repeated back for the rest of the group what he was hearing, "Yeah, you can't get better on three squares of shit food."

With people on the margins, and even with people who have enough money to buy good food, talking about grams or micrograms of vitamins, or food servings recommended for their health, or the upper limits of sugar and salt is not generally helpful. Thus, if I could ask a second question to assess your eating patterns, it would be, "*Where did the food from your last meal come from*?"

Our health is intimately connected with the health of our neighbors and our land. Many farmworkers who tend fields and animals are not treated fairly, nor paid equitably. In our eagerness to pull as much food from the earth as cheaply as possible, soil can be left depleted. The nutrients that plants draw from the soil must be replaced in the natural cycle of decomposition of food scraps and other organic matter.

Who it is that prepares our food should also be a consideration. There is a strong correlation between homemade meals and health—really, between eating out frequently and poorer nutritional status. Food made at home tends to be made with more wholesome ingredients, and, as we cook with others, we share invaluable skills and cultural knowledge.

When someone, especially a marketer, refers to *healthy* food, they usually mean what is healthy for our bodies, particularly what is *healthy* for our tummy paunches. But what if we defined food as *healthy* only if those who grew, tended, processed, prepared and served it were healthy—as well as the dirt where the plants grew, and the water source near the farm? We are making significant steps towards more sustainable diets, but how often do we pop something in our mouths without considering the journey that food took before it reached us?

If allowed a third question to assess your diet, it would be, "*Did you say grace before eating?*" When we pause to express gratitude, or practice mindful eating, we acknowledge that the food we are about to eat is a precious gift—not to be taken for granted, but consumed with intentionality. We reflect on how our survival, and our flourishing, is dependent on a large network of systems, starting with the rising of the sun, and including the countless people who tended, processed and transported the food we are about to enjoy. We recognize that some food choices lead us to participate in often-destructive systems, and thus we give thanks with humility.

Those who gather around a table often have different understandings, if grace is said at all, of whom the prayer is directed to. My wise friend Karen has people around her table several nights a week. She starts each meal, not assuming that everyone present prays, but with such a gracious invitation to remember that we live in an overly-independent, isolated culture, and that the food before us reminds us of our connection to each other. Somehow, that reminder makes even simple meals taste better.

We also say grace to remind ourselves that we are participating in a celebration, no matter how meager the meal, sparking our imaginations to see new ways of honoring the miracles of life. Some of our First Nations neighbors traditionally offer a prayer for the spirit of the animal who gave its life for the feast about to be consumed. Before eating, Japanese people say *itadakimasu*, meaning, "I humbly receive this food."

I grew up in a family that was deliberate about saying grace before each meal, no matter where we ate. While this felt awkward when we were at a restaurant or when a friend from a different background joined us for a meal, I now appreciate the value of pausing with others to be thankful.

A neighbor invited me to dinner one evening. She is Japanese and a professional chef, so I knew I was in for a treat. I arrived at the invited time, and she ushered me to my seat at her table. She had prepared a number of different dishes, all artistically plated. I have a reasonably good knowledge of food, but I could only name about half of what I saw. I was unsure of how to approach a few of the items on the table, but I figured I could follow my host's lead.

We smiled politely at each other, and I tried my clumsy, "*Itadakimasu*." My neighbor responded with a phrase she had learned from my culture, "Dig in, please." Then she got up and returned to her kitchen. I did not catch what she said as she got up, but soon enough learned that it was something like, "I forgot the dish with the thinly sliced raw beef marinated in a lemony soya sauce, so I will get that now." Despite my misgivings, that dish was delicious.

As my neighbor was putting the garnish on her raw meat plate, I wondered if starting to dish up food for myself was rude or expected. In the culture I grew up in, the prayer was also the signal that we could start eating, and everyone should have the chance to do so together. She had invited me to start, but it felt wrong to do so before she sat down again.

If I could ask a fourth question to assess your nutrition status, it would be, "*Who sat at the table with you as you ate?*" Loneliness is recognized as one of the primary issues in Vancouver, and despite the availability of much good food, too many of our neighbors live in *deserts*, without adequate access to fresh food, or in a vacuum of human relationships. Eating alone is strongly correlated with depression and other acute mental health challenges. We are seeing more and more studies suggesting that even smoking is not as detrimental to our health and longevity as loneliness.

Our enjoyment of food comes from companionship experienced while sharing a meal, not just the taste or relief of hunger. Eating a meal with someone changes the dynamics of your relationship. Strangers are no longer strangers after you have shared food with them, especially if you washed your dishes together after eating.

I heard a speaker who had been invited to Vancouver to talk about how we can make this city healthier. I cannot remember much of what he said, except that he explained how he did a fair bit of traveling across the country, often flying in the evening before his meetings or presentations. He would try to go for a walk after settling into his hotel, and start to do a quick assessment of whatever neighborhood he had landed in by counting the number of people he saw walking, the number of trees he passed, and how easy it was to find a fresh apple. We create food deserts in cities, which makes it challenging to offer hospitality and get to know our neighbors.

Street Testing for Celiac

Thinking about what we should eat goes together with what we should not eat. Wheat, or gluten, certainly gets its share of attention. When I was a dietetics student in the late 1990s, a primary focus of my lessons was around fiber and all the good it does for us. Since then, fiber seems to have gone out of fashion, although the powers behind the internet assume I am interested in it. I see a lot of advertisements for bran cereals scroll down the sides of my screens. Before I knew about online cookies and targeted ads, I thought everyone saw the same commercials, and I was amazed at how much fiber was marketed.

The common secret to low-carb, high-protein, Paleo, Whole 30, or whatever other trend diet seems to make people feel better is, in large part, cutting down sugar, salt and fat (whichever fats we currently understand to be the *bad* ones). The other significant weight-stabilizing, appetite-moderating, mood-steadying, bowel-regulating, cancer-fighting benefit of trend diets comes simply from increasing our consumption of plants (fiber) that have not been ultra-processed.

I once received a request to see a client with a "wheat flour allergy." When I asked his parole officer what that meant, he said, "He's trying to be healthy. He's vegetarian and doesn't eat wheat." Regrettably, I did not have the time to explore how vegetarianism and wheat-free eating are not necessarily synonymous with being healthy, nor what other nutrition advice that parole officer might dispense.

When I got to ask the individual himself what he meant by his reported allergy, he said, "I'm pretty sure I'm celiac. I was tested on the street." I should have asked exactly what he meant by that, but I was distracted by images of someone in a grubby lab coat pulling out a needle, running blood samples though a bicycle-powered assay machine (again, this is Vancouver), and pronouncing the person who just handed over $200 to be *allergic*, or *intolerant*, or *sensitive*.

Because this image amused me, and I imagined a friend who works in the same neighborhood might need something to smile about, too, I sent her a text, asking if her department monitors unregulated, underground testing for celiac disease.

"I'll see if we can add it to the list!! Wow!" was her response.

"Alternately, if no departments monitor it, we can start street testing and fund our next extravagant holiday," I joked back. Really, it was a joke—although people *would* pay for it in a rash attempt to understand why our digestion, and thus whole body, heart and mind, feels off some days. But to be clear, street testing is probably not ethical, and I am not suggesting anyone pursue this.

My friend responded, "It is trendy! We could add other pseudo-science testing to the panel and get paid in second-hand methadone." Also a joke, although the underground market for methadone, meal-replacement drinks, and other food or substances is fascinating. I was once offered a lifetime supply of Honeycomb cereal for only $4 as I walked past an impromptu street vendor. It was really a family-sized box of cereal, but for me, it would have been a lifetime supply.

A Few Other Rules

People who live without adequate income and who have many pressing needs, like where to sleep that night and where to get clean skivvies, are not able to buy what it takes for balanced meals and good snacks. Nutrition talks for this population need to focus on basic self-care, and small things that will help them get though the next hours or days. "Just for today," is a common encouragement in the Alcoholics Anonymous circles, and thus it is where I start conversations about eating.

I often use the ideas of a hunger scale with images of Lego figures showing distress, milder discomfort, neutral emotion, happiness, discomfort, and again distress, corresponding with the hunger phases we pass through all day (ideally, avoiding the extreme ends): starving—hungry—neutral—satisfied—full—stuffed. Most of my clients seem to understand the emotions displayed and connect to the Lego figures.

It is a good tool to explain why we make particularly poor decisions at times, especially when we get closer to the starving end. Someone in a group often brings up the term *hangry*, which makes sense to most people, even if it is the first time they have heard the term. A hunger scale is also a good tool to respond to assertions like one should *never* eat after 8:00 pm. I hear all sorts of rules like that. I point back to the scale, saying that if we are at the hungry end of the continuum, having not eaten enough through the day, a snack is a good idea. It is difficult to relax and fall asleep if we are hungry, an experience that can be confirmed by most of my group members. If we are full enough, but we reach for a snack out of habit or boredom, that snack will push us too far to the right side of the scale, impacting our quality of sleep, as well as how well we do on the scale the next day, swinging back and forth.

The hunger scale is a way of talking about intuitive, mindful eating, a practice which others have written on eloquently and extensively. We were good at intuitive eating when we were toddlers (as long as we were not distracted by sweets), but if you do not know what it means now—if you struggle to eat when you are hungry, or stop when you are full, while balancing that with regular rhythms of meals, snacks, rest, and activity—then it might be worth putting this book down and picking up one on mindful eating.

Intuitive eating is easier to follow than strict diet plans, and because my crowd tends to be anti-authority and mistrustful of government publications (occasionally leaning towards fun conspiracy theories), I use those principles more than the Food Guide or other official templates, although I do have a few rules. I endorse many of Michael Pollan's Food Rules,[1] which are clever, adoptable and science-based, and can be summed up with, "eat food, not too much, mostly plants." While I remain a spirit-of-the-law kind of person, I do tend to stick to the following rules to the letter.

Rule #1—Do not eat anything with "surprise" or "delight" or "super-size" in its name, except for "Surprise-Delight," a one-pot meal that my friend Greg used to make (to lovingly challenge my boundaries), which consisted of a can of beans, a can of tomatoes, and whatever else was in our fridge that needed cooking up.

Rule #2—Do not satisfy hunger with something sweet. I often hear from program participants that they are hungry *all of the time*. If someone has not consumed enough in the season leading up to

1. Pollan, Michael. *Food Rules: An Eater's Manual.*

coming into a shelter or supportive program, he or she will crave sweet calories. Add to that the brain desiring the rewards that the substances were providing, plus exhaustion and the potential for a quick energy surge, and it is inevitable that someone would be drawn to sugar. But sweet foods tend to have fewer good nutrients, so consider cravings for sweets as a signal to eat a good snack, and save treat foods as a reward.

One afternoon, I received a text from a friend while I was at my desk: "I ate a big peanut butter rocky road square an hour ago and now I feel bad." I knew enough about her overall diet and activity to not be concerned about her health or any excessive guilt she might be feeling, but I could empathize with the sensations that come with overindulging post-lunch sugar cravings.

My response: "Drink some water, say a prayer of confession, find some stairs to walk up and down for a minute, and next time, save half of it for a buddy that might be coming by after work." I was planning on going to her place at the end of the day to make something for a birthday dinner we were both invited to that evening.

Her response: "Brilliant. Thank you for this dietitian confessional. Off to do penance. . ."

Rule #3—No chocolate before 10:00 am. This is partly because I do not prefer strong flavors in the morning, but mostly it is because it is important to eat something solid within a few hours of getting up. If we can eat our first meal before we get too hungry, it is easier to get into the rhythm of having something savory and higher fiber, and not indulge in sweet carbs, or at least it is helpful to get some of the healthier food servings in before delving into one's daily treat allotment (if only we could stick to that). In my line of work, I rarely suggest "breakfast," as many of my clients are out of the habit of good morning routines and can get overwhelmed with the idea of frying eggs, making oatmeal, squeezing oranges into juice and keeping all the ingredients on hand that one would need for what marketers tell us is a *healthy* breakfast.

Rule #4—Never serve anything you have not tasted. Especially if it was made by other cooks, and those cooks were the colorful volunteers or participants in your community food program. Such individuals, while keen, hard-working, and often competent cooks, have been known to generously over-spice stews and overheat thick sauces. The percentage of such willing cooks who smoke tends to be higher than the rest of the population, at least in health-conscious Vancouver, and the nicotine habit affects their taste buds.

Over-spicing can also happen because of the curious chemistry of upscaling food. A recipe for four servings cannot be translated into a recipe for 150 by multiplying every ingredient by 37.5. There is a science to large-scale recipe conversion, so one would be wise to batch cook or let yourself be discipled by a seasoned chef before attempting large meals.

There is also a risk of under-salting food, as salt sometimes has a worse reputation than it deserves. When I cook in programs where we make food from scratch, using few of the cans and packages found in the middle aisles of grocery stores that we are cautioned to limit, I often have to convince my volunteer cooks that a little salt will bring out a lot of flavor.

This rule also speaks to food safety. When we cook for others, especially those who are vulnerable, we need to be more conscientious than when we cook for ourselves at home. While I may use the same spoon to taste, adjust seasoning, stir and taste again for something I cook for myself, it is safer (and kinder) to use a newly washed spoon for each tasting when cooking for others. Hygienic food handling practices, while absolutely necessary, are sometimes overly emphasized, as I often have to encourage volunteer cooks to taste food as they go.

I forget that safe ways to cook are not as much part of everyone's core fiber. A client proudly told me one day that he had just passed a FOODSAFE course. Given his recent history, I knew that this was a significant accomplishment. As I congratulated him for his good work, I was about to make a comment about how the ideas in the course were mostly common sense when he said, emphatically, about what he had just learned, "Man, there is so much that I had no idea about!"

Rule #5—Train your taste buds. We will eat what we like and what is convenient, not what we know is healthy, especially when we are tired or stressed. Just like we can have a sweet (or salty) tooth, we can train ourselves to crave healthier food if we pay attention to how we feel after we eat good food (and the foods that are no so good for us). This takes deliberate planning and intentionality, but it is possible to change our tastes for the better, and to help those in our care do the same.

Rule #6—Keep food simple so you can focus on hospitality. Set the table and put food into beautiful serving dishes. We eat first with our eyes, and presentation makes a difference to how much we eat, and how nourished we feel by our meal. I learned this lesson first from my mom, and then from Mona, a volunteer I have been fortunate enough to work with in several local programs. Both make a regular practice of putting flowers on the tables when we serve guests, or beautiful leaves and branches in the winter months. The flip side of this idea is that, when preparing food for others, we can get too caught up in making food look right, and forget to engage those who are in the room with us, or not allow our guests the joy of participating in the process.

Whether you are having one person at the table with you, or planning for a large community feast, the setting matters. It is as important as what we eat.

Parachute Meals

I have had a number of conversations over the years with friends and colleagues who are in the midst of organizing a group of their friends, family, students, staff, or volunteers to make a stack of sandwiches, cookies, and hot chocolate, or some variation on that menu. On a cold winter's night, the group will bundle up, drive to the poorer part of town, hand out their meals, chat with a few of the undernourished recipients, then drive home and feel good about what they did. These kinds of activities with a group are fun, at least for the sandwich givers, but do we consider how they feel for the recipients? How do they look from a larger food-systems and community-building perspective? Food-drops, or parachute meals, can feel shaming for those on the receiving end, especially if individuals do not get an opportunity to reciprocate the kindness. It does not usually feel as good to receive as it does to give.

There are many acute needs for food, and times when giving out a meal is a way to care for vulnerable people. For groups who do want to plan a meal to give out on the streets, take extra precautions around the safety and appropriateness of the food you serve. There will likely be people in the lineup with poor teeth or food intolerances, who have to face, again, the choice between hunger and food that will make them feel almost as bad as an empty stomach. Be especially sensitive if you film or take pictures of yourself or one of the recipients.

Such activities tend to be high waste, with the food packaging and unwanted parts of the meal tossed out. As Vancouver (and beyond) moves toward zero-waste, we should be prioritizing more hospitable shared meals without single-use dishes. We will return to the idea of food charity and creation care later.

Here are some alternate suggestions to care for our vulnerable neighbors. First, question why we would do anything if it does not involve sitting down with people, learning names, listening, and sharing stories. Partner with one of the amazing organizations or people in the neighborhood who work year-round to build relationships and support individuals on the margins, and ask what specific needs they have. If your group has a particular concern for a vulnerable sub-population—people in recovery, at-risk youth, seniors, women, families, new immigrants—ask about programs for such individuals. Groups can also collect socks, basic hygiene items, and gently used warm clothing. Single items are usually more helpful than predetermined care packages.

Supportive organizations are often swamped with volunteers and donations around Christmas, and experience a slump in the early part of the new year (and often in late summer). Spread your generosity through the whole year.

And finally, we must reiterate that it is only when someone has a home and an adequate income will he or she be food secure and cease experiencing acute hunger and its complications. Advocate for poverty reduction and supportive housing programs.

A healthy diet is not just the food and nutrients we put into our bodies, but the many ways we care for ourselves, and those around us. Before exploring more of the complexities of food programs, we will look at self care, and what makes such an essential practice so difficult.

Chapter 3

Self Care

Prison Might be a Nice Break

"I DON'T KNOW HOW you do this week after week, Karen." Guests at the community meals occasionally make comments like this, and it always surprises me. I also hear, "I won't be at the dinner tomorrow at your church, I need to take a day off, I'm burned out," from my usual guests when I run into them at other community events. Undernourished people are often at a point of low resilience, drained by the more-than-full-time work of finding food and by the presence of so many others in a similar state.

Imagine having not slept properly last night, maybe for several nights, having an uncontrollable set of hormones raging through your body, commanding you to EAT SOMETHING NOW. Imagine you feel some social anxiety, or at least are in the mood to eat in the company of a small group of trusted friends, not two hundred near strangers. Maybe you are craving protein, or your stomach is feeling off from a bug you picked up, and you have mostly eaten highly processed, low fiber foods, which are not gentle on your digestive system. All this adds up to craving, and deserving, a good meal in a peaceful setting.

The stress of sustained poverty makes it nearly impossible to care for oneself. In one group nutrition session, a man with diabetes explained his condition, and he seemed to have a general understanding of the impact of what he ate on his body's ability to regulate his blood sugars—but then he said, "When I feel the shakes [from low blood sugar], and I stuff my face with doughnuts, I feel better. So what should I stuff my face with?"

While I considered how to respond to that, another guy in the group said, "Dude, that's your problem, I think. Probably we aren't supposed to stuff our faces." Then he turned to me and asked, "Is that right?" so earnestly that I could only nod and affirm his advice.

So, how do I sustain myself? How do I ensure I never get to a place where stuffing a few doughnuts into my mouth will make me feel better than my current state?

Sometimes I don't. Sometimes I dream of having a job where I do not get my hands so dirty, do not have to call 9-1-1, or do not have to rescue a big batch of cornbread from a distracted volunteer who put too much baking soda into the batter, though I at least now know how to address that problem. If you ever find yourself with just a little too much baking soda in a recipe, add some lemon juice or vinegar. If there is more than twice the amount of baking soda than was called for, scrap what you have and start again. Whatever you are baking will not taste right in the end.

During one particularly busy season, a man at one of my community meals told me he had a two-year jail sentence waiting for him in the United States, and he was trying to work up the courage to turn himself in and get it over with. My first thought was, "Prison might actually be a nice break for a while." I put in a vacation request that afternoon.

I am getting better at realizing when I am doing too much, stretching myself too thin. My Mennonite heritage, Enneagram score, and basic temperament all lead me to love cooking for others, and be generous with what I have. If I want a cup of tea, which is a reality once or twice a day, I assume that whoever else is in the room with me also wants tea, and I will offer to make two cups.

But, when I do too much, I begin to lose all inclination towards generosity. It starts small—I will be washing my mug, and will see another one sitting beside the sink. My hands are already wet, and it would be no more effort to wash that one too, but I cannot bring myself to do so. Or when someone at a community dinner asks for a pair of socks, and I know there is a bin full of new socks that were donated for people like him, but my first reaction is to hang on to those socks, I know I need to feed my heart a little more.

So I eat breakfast. Literally. Liberally. If we have been fasting for ten hours or so, we need to fuel our bodies well before we can act well, think well, move well, love well. Not eating enough in the first half of the day is one of the bigger nutritional mistakes many people make. We get busy, fill up on caffeine, do not make the time to plan good snacks, and then get too hungry later in the day. This makes us do things we would not normally do—eat an excess of cheap snacks, snap at someone, get clumsy and stub a toe, or forget something important. What matters, really, is not so much when we eat, but how that adds up in a day, or over a few days, but eating earlier in the day usually gives us more sustained mental and physical energy.

I try to feed my spirit breakfast, too. I start most mornings with a cup of tea and a book, nothing electronic. I read stories of people who have started food and shelter programs, people who have come through addictions and mental illness, articles about different ways of looking at the world, and, occasionally, even The Good Book. I look for stories of people who have found the balance between contemplation and action, or sometimes stories of people who drastically lost that balance. The quietness nourishes me, as well as the insights others articulate.

I also get to witness resurrection in many small ways, which sustains me as much as any meal. I met Jack, a guest at one community meal, when he had a full, unkempt beard. After he had volunteered with us for nearly a year, I got to compliment him the first day he shaved it off. "I don't need my shield anymore," he said. I knew a guy who went by Shadow, but with a group where he belonged, he allowed us to call him by his given name, William. I knew a man who introduced himself as MatthewMarkLukeAnd-John. When he healed and stabilized enough, he remembered his name was just Luke.

"I believe in God," I read with Sharyn, a dear friend standing beside me, and with a hundred strangers, in a beautiful old church in New York City. "I believe in . . . the resurrection of the body." We were in the Central Presbyterian Church, built in the 1920s by the Rockefeller family, and for almost a century, kindred spirits had been gathering every Sunday morning, learning how to sustain themselves. I had three weeks of holidays, and I knew I needed to spend some time outside of a big city, but I first wanted to visit Sharyn and experience the energy of New York. In that moment, I was encouraged by how I could show up anywhere in the world, find a church, and feel a connection with others who are also learning to practice resurrection.

Sustaining oneself has to include an intentional practice and frequent experiences of gratitude. When I can find a few minutes to stand at the exit door and say *good-bye* as guests leave community meals, I receive many *thank you*'s. I re-realized the value of this when I was visiting a community meal where the volunteers were all busy cleaning up as the guests finished their meal and left. I noticed several people pause at the door, seemingly looking for someone to thank, but no one was there.

Halfway through my undergrad degree, when funds were low, I shared a room with Kate. We actually shared a bunk bed, which gave us space for two desks in a room in a shared house, making our rent low enough to fit our student budgets. Out of a spirit of generosity for our new friendship, I offered to take the top bunk, though it would be a hassle every time I wanted to get in and out of bed. Kate, similarly, offered to take the lower bunk, thinking she was offering me the privilege of the better bed. Fortunately, honesty won over Canadian politeness, and we sorted out our preferred layers.

Inspired by Oprah Winfrey, Kate made us both little gratitude journals, and for several months, we wrote down five things for which we were grateful before going to sleep. On the nights I did not feel like it, or could not muster up the energy to be grateful for anything, Kate would jump down from her bunk and make up some things for me, her name usually making it onto my gratitude list. I have not kept up the daily journal, but have returned to it in different seasons.

My energy to reflect at the end of most days is limited, but I have found one practice I can follow. The Examine is the practice of articulating the three most life-giving and three most draining things from each day. It helps to see that no matter how tough a day was, there are at least three things that I am grateful for. And that the three hardest things in my day can be given over to The Sustainer, who cares about the intricate details of life. For a season, another friend, also Kate, and I emailed this to each other at the end of every day. Having someone to receive it was helpful.

Whenever I sit down to a meal with my nieces, everyone at the table is invited to express gratitude for something. One day, Belle, aged three, must have been miffed at being called away from her toys or because she was strongly encouraged to put a shirt on for dinner, as her prayer was, "Dear Jesus, thank you for nothing!" Her dad and I tried not to laugh as we said what we felt thankful for, but I had to admire the kid's honesty. In that moment, she could not see how many good things she had in her life, but she knew how to express what her heart was feeling. I must admit also to moments of struggling to feel gratitude for all that is on my plate, but when I take time to reflect, I recognize there is an abundance to be thankful for.

Part of realistic self care is reminding oneself regularly that we are no one's savior. Although I believe the community meals I am connected with are significant, people will survive without me. Jesus, I am sure, felt plenty of pressure to do more good things, but he knew his human body and his crew needed downtime. I have heard a theory that Jesus was likely an INFJ (Introversion, Intuition, Feeling, Judging) on the Myers-Briggs personality chart. I use this as my working theory, since I have the same personality traits, and like to imagine what he needed to do to restore himself.

Humility + A Strong Will

Somewhere I read of a review of the personalities of individuals who had turned struggling organizations into successful ones. The two traits they shared were humility and a strong will. This has stayed with me, as I had thought it was more front-of-the-crowd oration skills that inspired action, but I have come to see that the leaders I admire do have these qualities. Luckily, I was born with a wee stubborn streak, and I get humbled all the time.

A few years ago, Jo, a woman who works in *lifestyle TV*, felt convicted when the world was facing the crisis of the Syrian refugees. She realized she was having fun with her creative, professional skills, but that they were having no impact on people who were struggling around the world. Her friends suggested she look into local hunger and food insecurity. She found a group I was working with and offered to donate her time, and the time of some talented colleagues, to make a video.

We recognized this was a gift far beyond what our budget could otherwise afford. A good storyteller could help us show how hunger affects more people in cities like Vancouver than most of us realize; and how small, regular community kitchens, or cooking groups, are one of the simplest ways to foster relationships, share food, and develop the agency that will give individuals the resilience to address the challenges of poverty. Together, we came up with a script that would tell this story in about five minutes, found a venue, invited some program participants, and I pulled up a menu from a previous community kitchen I had run.

The filming was set for a few days before Cinco De Mayo, one of my favorite holidays, being a day to remember an unlikely victory in Mexico, a day to honor the personalities of Japanese children, a day to celebrate the birth of significant historical figures such as Karl Marx and Soren Kierkegaard, and my own birthday. Everyone I have influence to feed, which is really a lot of people, eats Mexican food in early May. I planned for us to make fish tacos, a meal that is colorful, tasty, can keep many hands busy with different items to chop, does not have long cooking times, is *West-Coast-ish*, and would be a fit for whatever vegan-kosher-gluten-free-or-other special dieters might show up. Plus, the meal could include beans, which would help me live up to the reputation I once earned of being fervently committed to "food, justice and plant-based proteins."

We had a good turnout that day and meal prep started well. I knew many of the participants, though it was my first time meeting Janice, an older Danish woman who wore such vibrant sparkly green eye shadow that I wondered if anyone standing beside her would look ghostlike in the footage. We got a team set up to make ginger-mint fruit salad, another making coleslaw, and a few others making black bean salsa. Thankfully, I got gloves on my boss just before he helpfully started chopping jalapeño peppers for the first time, so he would not curse me later when spicy capsicum compounds were burning his fingertips. All that was left was the fish.

Janice and I read over the recipe. While our salmon fillets were defrosting, I CLEARLY explained that we would make a coating for the fish of flour, baking soda, and chili powder. THEN we would make a marinade of lime juice, salt, sugar, and a little more chili powder. We would marinate the fish, dip it in the coating, and then cook it.

We made the flour coating, and I suggested Janice start on the marinade while I got the fish. When I turned back to her three seconds later, she had added the lime juice to the flour mixture, and it was bubbling up and over the bowl, the acid from the limes reacting to the baking soda in the flour mixture.

"Oh, we didn't want to mix those," I tried to say gently, not wanting to make her feel bad for taking some initiative, while attempting to rewrite the recipe in my head and figure out how to rescue the meal. The ingredients would all go into the same dish in the end, but the texture would not be the same. Dousing a foamy white volcano while responding to Janice's profuse apologies was not the image of myself that I wanted on video. We scrapped the flour coating, found another seasoning for the fish, and got it in the oven. When rolled up in the tortillas, it tasted just fine.

More Acts of Sustenance

To sustain myself and replenish my energy to enter some chaotic and challenging settings, I also carve out time for creativity. I need to make things beautiful, just for beauty's sake, for creation's sake. We eat first with our eyes. I have written two children's books, each a gift for my nieces who pop up in these pages, two delightful souls who could be the central characters in a number of good stories. The books are also creative expressions of what I learn at work. The first, called *Two Soups in One Day*, is about one of the most fundamental things that any of us can do to care for ourselves and our communities—cook good food from scratch and share it with someone. The second, called *Myself Today*, is about what erodes and restores resilience. I was fortunate enough to connect with two great artists, whose drawings made the characters and ideas come to life.

My sustenance rituals also include keeping reminders that I am loved. I get a letter from my mom every week or two with newspaper clippings of interest. After being introduced once, my new acquaintance said to me, "Oh, you're a dietitian. You must know a lot of interesting facts." I had not known that is what a dietitian's reputation was built on, but any interesting facts I know are as much from my mom's envelopes as from any classes I have taken. And I am reminded that I am loved when my dad is genuinely delighted *every time* I call or walk through their door.

Or I remember a tiff with Kate when we shared that bunk bed while at university. The fight was about whether we would buy cheaper eggs, which were at least from my hometown, Abbotsford, an hour away, or the most expensive eggs, which advertised letting the chickens roam free in their yard. As a student, I could not justify my limited budget being splurged on chicken freedom, but it mattered to Kate. We argued about it, I went out, we both fumed, and when I got back home later that night, Kate was asleep, but there was a note next to my bed saying, "G, I made you an egg salad sandwich for your lunch tomorrow. It is in the fridge." She had bought eggs and made me a lunch, knowing I would be on campus all day. I do not know what emotional state the chickens that laid those eggs were in, but when I eat egg salad sandwiches, I still think about her simple-silly act of forgiveness, care and sustenance.

Or I remember going to visit my friend Juliette, a recent refugee from Burundi who was now living here in Canada with her three young children. The youngest, Marvilles, at five years old, had more spirit in his wiggly little body than most people I know combined. Walking up to their house one day, he saw me approaching and ran out his front door, then launched himself off the steps, exclaiming, "Karen! I love you! I missed you! Catch me!"

Or I remember my niece Elli sitting down beside me on her daddy's front porch as I was blowing bubbles with her. "Aunt," she said, with all the adoring earnestness that a little kid can muster, "I want to be like you." What I think she meant as she put her hand on mine was, "I want that bubble wand that you are currently in possession of, and I want to be able to create magical, shiny soap spheres as big as yours," but it makes me smile to remember it. And I need that in the midst of a pile of dirty dishes and volunteers disagreeing about whose responsibility they are.

My community supports me when I need it. The first time Vancouver's overdose crisis got too close, and I watched life slip out of a man right outside the doors of a community lunch I coordinated, I was affected deeply. His name was Jordan, and he had been an occasional guest at my program. It happened on the same day that our good neighbors to the south bewilderingly elected Mr. Trump to be their next president. Jordon's passing did not generate as many headlines, or any that I could find, but his life made an impact. As I write this, some time has passed, but I can recognize that I still do not have the same buoyancy as I did before Jordan's death. I am a little more tired, inside and out, and things that I normally enjoy, like a few minutes of quality time with *The National* at the end of the day, I cannot face right now. I grew up with the voice of Knowlton Nash, then CBC's main anchor, as the background to my bedtime routine, and then for many years it was Peter Mansbridge. I miss him now that he has retired.

As paramedics attempted to save Jordan, I stepped outside to see if I could talk to his friend, trying to imagine how she was feeling as she helplessly watched this horrific scene unfold. I asked if I could sit next to her, and when she said yes, I learned that she goes by Tony, short for Antoinette. Tony was staying in the shelter a few blocks away. Most of her family was still in northern Manitoba. She had not known Jordan well, but they had forged a street friendship. He would just pop up unexpectedly, she told me with a wistful smile. Tony had made it partway through her training to be a Red Seal Chef. She did not say that she dropped out of school because of an addiction, but I guessed from her appearance that was likely the case. Green curries were her specialty, though she liked the challenge of improvising recipes from whatever she would find in the fridge. I told her she would fit right in with our community meal team and got another sad smile.

Several police officers came by to ask Tony questions, and through it all, my volunteer team amazingly pulled the meal together. Even crusty old Larry, who was six days clean at that point, and probably in some pain, and who was often quick to express his disapproval of any women in leadership or government action, came over with two cups of coffee for Tony and me. Larry had added way more sugar than I prefer, but Tony seemed to appreciate it. On another day, I might have explored with Larry how to change his taste for coffee to be less sweet, but this was not the time. I was just grateful for his thoughtful way of checking in with me.

I wrote of Jordan's passing and my fatigue to my longtime friend Sarah, whose path took her to the UK. I got this back, and have re-read it many times since then, whenever I need encouragement, or find myself exhausted:

> *hello, my dear friend—ugh. i'm sorry—empathetically so—about your week. many of us are grieving over the stories of hate and fear that are springing up everywhere in the aftermath of the US elections, but your personal experience of death literally on your doorstep brings a sense of hopelessness directly into the heart of it . . . you're real about it—it being both the love of God and the sometimes*

crappy and sometimes beautiful realities in which we live. i'll try and remember to pray tomorrow morning as you prepare for your day and week and try and shape some story of hope amidst the rubble in your communities. go in peace, dear karen—sarah

Or I remember walking through Main & Hastings on my way to work one morning—one of the most notorious intersections in Vancouver, where low voices whisper offers of a good deal on cigarettes, blocks of cheddar cheese, Tylenol 3's, Percocet's, marijuana, and increasingly harder substances. It was one of the first nice spring mornings, and I made eye contact with a haggard-looking gentleman. He said something about the weather, and then something about my smile. Another guy then rode his bike up onto the curb, and I had to jump back to avoid getting run over. The first man then said, "Be careful, Miss. You are way too precious to lose."

Unexpected Surprises

And some days, I am renewed by unexpected surprises. One morning I was sitting quietly at my desk, trying to put together a newsletter, stewing about how someone had not yet finished a piece he said he would write, when my phone rang. It was Lee. Since the stay in the hospital when she had befriended the dominatrix, Lee had spent more time on the streets, and now was in a different hospital. Skipping the usual hello-how-are-you, she launched with, "Remember we said it would happen fast, remember we prayed for a place? It already happened, I'll need some things for my room, I'm in a house with people who are already stabilized." I have a pile of prayers that do not seem to get answers, but some days, hardened homeless women teach us that the important prayers do get heard. That one was especially beautiful, because the collective faith that she and I had when we prayed for a home for her during our last conversation was so small that I cannot even think of an apt metaphor.

It took a few months before I made the trip out to visit Lee in her new facility, but when her birthday came, I promised to take her to dinner. She chose The Keg, and despite my New Year's resolution that year to lean more vegan, and a budget that did not allow for many steak dinners, I figured she deserved to be treated, so we went and had a lovely meal. When I tried to pay for it, the waitress told me that the man who had been sitting at the next table over had paid our bill when he left a few minutes before. Lee does not have an inside voice, and the man must have overheard much of our conversation, and picked up on her history. It was such a cool surprise.

Finding the Extra Reserves

"Hey, Karen, a guy called Hank wants to talk to you," one of my volunteers said at the end of a community dinner. I was in the hallway, debriefing with a few others about how the evening had unfolded. We were in the midst of transitioning from an overcrowded lineup to a café-style meal, with fewer tables and chairs set up, food available for longer, and waiters who take orders and bring customized plates based on limited choices, but at least some choice.

Hank could be unpredictable, and would likely ask for something I did not have to offer. At that moment, I was emotionally done, a reaction I recognized I was having more often in those days.

Resisting the urge to slip out the back door, go home, curl up in my favorite chair, and find a detective drama, I reached down into my well of reserve energy, and walked to the dining hall, which was empty, except for one volunteer who was sweeping, and Hank, standing by a table in the corner. Unexpectedly, he launched into something like, "This is all too much, I don't know if I can take it anymore, it just hurts, I do not want to be here, I'm 52 and should have done more by now. Doctors keep prescribing me drugs, but they don't even take them to know what they feel like, and I hate going to the clinic for Methadone every day. I'm sorry I am crying." All that was laced with some rather creative uses of words that my mother would not approve of. I wondered how much more unrestrained the speech would have been if Hank had not just eaten a full meal. Or how else he might have expressed that pain if we had not held him in our community during the previous few hours.

I guided Hank towards a couch in the corner of the room, sat down next to him, and put my arm on his shoulders as he cried. Although we all need touch, it is generally not a good idea to initiate or allow physical contact with the people who come through community programs. We make that clear to new volunteers, but you eventually learn when touch is okay, and even necessary. Hank, at that moment, needed human contact. I suppose I did, too.

Once Hank's tears had been shed, he told me about how his wife had died five years ago, and he was still grieving, though he could not articulate it was grief that was weighing so heavily in that moment. He was also concerned for Paul, a guy who was squatting with him, a stray cat, and a clan of rats in the parkade across the street. I had sat in the exact same place with Paul a few weeks earlier as *his* story spilled out, bringing him near tears several times. The volunteer who had been sweeping came over to ask a question, and I asked her if she would get us some Kleenex. I learned later that she had thought I had asked for peanuts, and she had performed a thorough search of the storeroom for nuts before realizing what Hank had really needed.

After listening to what was weighing on Hank, we made a plan for him to come in early the next morning. We would set him up for a shower, then put him to work at the next meal. As he got up, Hank said, "Okay. Thanks. I should go now. Unless you want to go get a beer with me." I declined, telling him I was done for the day. He asked how long it took to put the meal on, seemingly realizing for the first time how much work was done before guests like him showed up to eat.

The next day, Hank did show up, three hours after he had said he would, buzzing like a bombed bumblebee. We got him a plate of food, and he ate a few bites, then got up and cleared some dishes. Then another bite of food, and he started collecting the water jugs on the tables. I explained that the meal was still on for another half hour, and we needed to put the water jugs back. We were trying to create a café-type atmosphere, and needed the tables to look neat and consistent.

"But no one is sitting at that table," Hank protested.

"People will come," my logic not getting through to him, but my will was stronger, so we put the water jugs back on the tables, and I led Hank back to his lunch. A few minutes later, he was up, again, folding and stacking chairs. I explained that the meal was still on for another twenty-five minutes, and we needed to put the chairs back.

"But no one is sitting at that table," Hank protested, again.

"People will come," my logic still not getting through to him, my patience coming from a source other than my natural inclination.

Facilitating Self Care

Teaching basic nutrition and meal service is less about food groups or what we understand this month about our daily requirements for vitamins, minerals, and other micronutrients. We find good eating patterns when we listen to and care for our bodies, and pay attention to the connections between what we put in our mouths and overall quality of life—both ours and other people who are involved in our food system.

I try to endorse the exact opposite approach as Sam, a client who dropped into my office at a treatment center to talk about what he could eat while he was there, given that he had diabetes, and had not been eating well during the last season of his life. "I'm going to lose my legs someday anyway, so I just eat what I want. Yesterday I had a Slurpee." I tried to not look troubled by his admission, and asked what he did when he experienced a low blood sugar swing. "Oh, I don't get those. I don't like how those feel, so I keep my blood sugars at 10 to 15." The normal range is 4 to 7 millimoles per liter. Anything higher than that can cause small blood vessels to burst, leading to irreversible damage.

Caring for oneself is impossible without a home, a place to be secure. "I'm brushing my teeth regularly for the first time in twenty years. And sleeping on a real bed," someone told me as he was just getting back on his feet. I do not feel right if I go more than half a day without brushing my teeth. Statements like this get to me viscerally.

Because I am so immersed in cooking and sharing food, I forget what is or is not common knowledge, or that there is such a range of what practices are innate, depending on the setting someone grew up in. One client acknowledged to me that he recognized that he did feel better, that his emotions, energy, thoughts, and sleep patterns were all more steady than they had been before he moved into the facility, and he recognized that this was in part because he was consistently eating healthy, varied meals and snacks each day. "But who does that?" he asked. "Who has time to make regular meals?" He had never experienced a rhythm of breakfast, lunch, and dinner. I was tempted to reply, "I do. And most healthy, sober people," but that might not have helped.

These practices, and many others, nourish us holistically. But one aspect of our self that needs particular care is our spirituality, which the next chapter will explore.

Chapter 4

Spirituality

Connected to Something Larger

Trying to take my faith into my work settings, my professional self into my faith settings, and carving out a life that has the same rootedness as I had growing up, yet makes sense in my adult world, made me realize at times, that I could not articulate what *faith* and *spirituality* really meant to me. What I had known when I was younger did not all feel true anymore, and I could no longer engage with many aspects of local church culture. Still, there remains an intangible chord that I choose to hang on to.

Judy Graves, one of Vancouver's more inspiring advocates, said in a radio interview with the CBC around the time of her retirement:

> I'll be retiring from the bureaucracy, but I won't be retiring from the people on the street. I can't. . .. I'm thankful for the gift that people have shared their stories with me, and enriched my life, my understanding of our city, of our world, of God. . .. My work has been my spiritual practice. . .. If you have to do your faith instead of talking about it, you can't kid yourself.

I have returned to Judy's comments often, hoping that I will be able so say something similar when I retire, and learn to have even half her eloquence. In a talk she gave to some medical professionals, she started by saying something like, "My friends frustrate you guys, and drive you crazy. But its okay. You're even. You frustrate them and drive them crazy, too."

A friend recently asked if I had found my tribe here in Vancouver, and I could say that I had. I have learned more about faith and grace in gritty food programs than I ever did on Sunday mornings in church services. I often find it hard to engage with sermons or communal singing, but sitting with someone who smells of stale _________ (pick your vice—cigars, pot, liquor, toothbrushlessness, shower aversion), fatigued by poverty, someone who has known chronic hunger, reminds me why the gospel matters.

The definition of spirituality that makes most sense to me is the realization that we are connected to something larger than ourselves. That is how spirituality is understood in the recovery community, and although I have not struggled with an addiction, at least not substance abuse, the accepting, lifeline spirituality I learn from my newly sober friends is what my faith needed to relearn what I grew up knowing.

We are wired for safety and connection. Through that lens, spirituality comes from practices that connect us to our Creator and our neighbors, and hopefully helps make faith communities safer places. It is the practices that root us and remind us we are kin. Such practices remind us that people act in ways that are reasonable to them, and that we can love those who seem to be acting unreasonably because we were first loved abundantly.

Our First Nations neighbors teach us the concept of the medicine wheel. We have physical, mental, emotional, and spiritual selves which are distinct, yet intimately connected. For health and healing, these four elements have to be in balance. I try to articulate examples of that balance being restored, especially where spirituality is not commonly part of the conversation.

A man I knew as Bill started a conversation at a community dinner one day by thanking me for helping him keep his apartment six months earlier. He had been on the verge of losing it, and I had printed off some forms for him. I had not done much, but it had helped him address a system that would too easily allow him to become homeless. It had only taken me a few minutes to find the forms he needed online, and I could easily do so because I had learned to navigate websites and had access to a functional printer. For someone on the edge, these little things can be the nudge that tips them over, that catastrophically unbalances the four selves.

Later, as we chatted while eating our dinner, Bill reflected, "I see tonight for the first time that we are really a community, not just a bunch of unlucky transients."

> Working with people who struggle, sometimes feels like not much changes, yet, because we are in close relationship, we know . . . they have felt loved and accepted, even if that feeling comes and goes. . .. [T]hey are giving to others, instead of only taking, they are experiencing less shame this year than last year. . .. If we remain so intertwined with people's hearts and stories that we notice each shift toward good instead of evil, light instead of darkness, hope instead of despair, we will find reason after reason to celebrate. The more we celebrate, the more God-at-work we seem to notice.

I copied that excerpt from *Down We Go* by Kathy Escobar[1] into my journal next to a recipe for crepes. I had been visiting a friend who made a breakfast of delicately thin pancakes that were above par. The secret, I learned, is to let the batter sit for at least a half hour before cooking. In the same way that the flour slowly interacts with the milk and eggs, it took that weekend getaway to help me to see the little shifts towards light that my hungry friends and I were experiencing.

Poor in Spirit

Another angle on spirituality, particularly poignant in the contexts I find myself in, is the degree that we learn to be *poor in spirit*.

1. Escobar, *Down We Go*, 217.

Scripture says we are blessed when we get there, but it is a concept that I still struggle to comprehend. I understand that it is good when we are humble enough to ask for help. Those who walk the Alcoholics Anonymous path embody this well, having learned to accept that they are powerless over something that controls them, and it is not their own strength that will help them through difficult circumstances.

Community meals taught me another translation for *poor in spirit*. If Jesus had used the food programs in Vancouver as the context in which to give us the Beatitudes, he might have said, "Blessed are those difficult volunteers who, whenever someone bumps into them, believe it was done intentionally, with malice, and who feel the need to make known to the program coordinator that they are being bullied, for those people who see themselves as victims will be shown grace, upon grace, upon grace, until their little hearts melt, and their little minds expand, and they become able to interpret a bump as nothing more than a miscalculation of spatial awareness."

It is almost amazing how often I find myself in the midst of a busy meal, listening to one of my crew explain how another person went out of their way to bump into them. One day, it was Julie. She had been volunteering with us for a few months, and had let me know multiple times that she was recovering from a brain injury. She could be helpful, but she did not seem to get many of the routines we were trying to put in place with our serving and cleaning up. Since Julie's tenure began, I had already had a few conversations with other volunteers who were frustrated with her for doing something *wrong*, or for telling them off. I would try to explain why it was important to make space for Julie, and that it was her brain injury, not a mean personality, that was causing the challenges.

I was in the midst of my own lunch, a yam and peanut soup, upcycled from the yam stew we had served the day before. We had made a pretty good soup by adding a little broth to the stew and whirring it up with our immersion blender (one of my favorite kitchen tools). We supplemented that with a spinach salad (compliments of a Mennonite church that had leftover greens from an event a few days before) and bagels (overstock from a new bagelry nearby).

While I was eating, Marcus sat down next to me. He is a rather nice looking man in his late fifties, clean and clean cut. He is courteous, quick to smile (showing off noticeably nice teeth), generally kind, and much less colorful than my average guest, both in personality and dress, though for the last few weeks he had been wearing a sling on his arm. As Marcus waited for his lunch, he told me in great detail about how he had ridden the bus to the church, and had been bumped, *intentionally*, by a series of ill-mannered people.

I did not feel like engaging with Marcus and his complaints, but I did intend to as I finished my lunch. Halfway through our meal, I got up to check on something, and Julie pulled me aside and told me that Marcus had walked a wide, unnecessary arc across the room a few minutes ago, just so he could rudely bump into her. She even demonstrated, by smashing her hip into mine, how the bump had felt, as she explained that she did not deserve to be bullied.

I affirmed that we shared an anti-bullying stance, then tried to get Julie to see if there might be another, more positive lens through which she could look at Marcus. Maybe he had not seen her. Maybe he was in pain himself.

"Oh, that sling he's wearing? It's fake! He says his arm was twisted by the police. That's not true. I've seen him use his arm," Julie pronounced, loud enough for Marcus to hear if he was paying attention to us, though he did not appear to be.

I tried my next tactic, which usually works, though it was less successful with Julie. "We run this meal so people who do not fit in anywhere else have a place to belong, and we are intentionally more tolerant here than other places we go." When I say that, I am frequently referring to the individual I am speaking with, as much as the person they are complaining about, but I suspect that the person I am with rarely sees that. And I explained, not for the first time, that, as a church volunteer, I did not expect Julie to hold to all the beliefs of the church, but I did expect her to show more grace here than she might elsewhere.

"But I am being bullied. Are you saying I shouldn't be here?" Julie threw back at me.

"No, Julie. You are a valuable part of this team." I hoped that I sounded more sincere than I felt. It would have been more honest to tell her she was more work than help, but I had earnest intentions to want her to feel like she was part of the team. Just by being born human, she was valuable. The same was true for Marcus. By this time, though, Julie had adopted a very defensive posture, and I was trying not to do the same.

I tried another angle, encouraged by a few guests who had finished their meal and walked a wide arc around the room to pass by me and thank me for lunch. This time, I evoked the wisdom of Brené Brown.[2] "Do you think Marcus is doing the best he can?" I asked Julie.

"Absolutely not," she shot back at me, without even pausing to consider what life was like for Marcus. I knew that Julie lived in North Vancouver, and Marcus lived a few miles south of the church, and I wondered how often they had run-ins. "I can see that I'm not appreciated here. I'll just go!" I did not have the energy or the wisdom to argue with her further.

Julie never did return to that program. It would have been at least a 45-minute ride on public transit to get to the church where the meal was hosted, and I wonder what had brought her there in the first place. Should I try to track her down and woo her back? Is she hurt and upset with me, or the church as a whole, or has she forgotten and connected elsewhere? Do she and Marcus realize that their attitudes leave people like me a little poorer in spirit after each conversation with them, needing a little more support from the rest of my community? How much does the network of compassionate programs in Greater Vancouver really impact people like Julie and Marcus—nourishing both body and spirit? These may be unanswerable questions, but worth pondering as we

2. Brown, *Rising Strong*.

set up, serve, and clean up our dinners, addressing all that arises in the process.

Scrunching Up & Grieving

"This is how I pray," said my niece Belle, aged three, just before lunch one day, scrunching her face up and pressing her little fists into her cheeks. She knew it was our tradition to have everyone at the table express thankfulness for something before we began to fill our plates. I am not sure if she was trying to rush the final dinner preparations, show off her new skill (we had taught her the word "scrunch" the day before when she realized she could manipulate many of her facial muscles), or if she had grasped that prayer is something worth putting our whole bodies into. "I hear you," I wanted to say. "That's how I feel, too."

That week, I had stopped at an art supplies store and bought a black portfolio-style book. Another church that runs a community meal has a memorial book that is pulled out when the community is processing the loss of someone, and it seemed time to set one up for the program I was working with.

We had heard a month ago that Rob Ferrier passed away, but I did not know how to verify if that was true. Rob had not visited our dinner for several weeks, though sporadic absences are not uncommon with this community. The individual who told me of Rob's passing had known him, and knew some other people in the building where he lived, so it was likely true, but I held on to hope that Rob would walk through our doors again. He had been an active volunteer with the meals long before I came around, having earned enough trust to get keys to the church. Rob was someone who saw little details like a splash of food dried on the wall, and would quietly take the time to scrub it off, not needing anyone to notice his work. He had *retired* from volunteering with us a few months earlier, though he still showed up most weeks to eat, hug me, and chat with his community. If we were short-handed, he would fill in where needed.

The closest I have ever come to smoking was an evening when I walked around the backside of the church building that hosted the dinner. Rob was peacefully watching the sunset with a lit cigarette in his mouth. It was Labour Day, and we had planned on having a BBQ outside, rather than set up tables and chairs inside like we usually did. We expected about one hundred people, but still planned enough food for our usual 150. Somehow, the word got out about the BBQ and well over 250 people showed up. A group had held a BBQ the day before at the church, so we delved into their leftovers once our food was gone. We still may have witnessed a miracle, as the food did not run out until everyone had a plateful, plus a second helping for the few hopefuls who hung around long enough.

Halfway through service, when our line of hungry people seemed longer than our stack of burgers, a nervous energy radiated from the crowd. Someone accused the guy in front of him of attempting to steal a jar of mustard, and that man took exception to the allegation. One person—I am not sure if it was the accuser or accused—threw a punch, and a lot of people started yelling. We got the situation resolved quickly enough, but it left me feeling on edge. When I was sure the risk of another altercation was minimal, I went to grab something from the kitchen. There were fewer doors to go through if I went around the outside of the building, and that is how I found Rob and his cigarette. I leaned into him as I told him about the mustard incident. He refused to let me have a cigarette, and I suppose I should remain grateful that he forced me to calm myself in other ways.

Rob had taken on the role of giving the church kitchen a thorough cleaning after the weekly meals. It is a thankless job that few people notice when it is done, but which many people comment on if not done. One week, after everyone but Rob had left, my colleague and I were in our office planning for the next week's meals, thankful for some quiet. Rob peeked in and said nonchalantly, "Can you do me a favor?" He did not ask for much, so I looked up expectantly and nodded as Rob carried a box into the office and set it down. He had bits of dirt and shrub all over him, as he had just crawled through the bushes outside the church to capture a duck with an injured wing. He set the duck in its box in the middle of the office and asked if we could find a vet that would help it. We called around and found a wildlife rescue center. My colleague was about to meet with another volunteer, so rather than sit in a café, they held their meeting as they drove the duck to the vet.

When I got confirmation that Rob had passed away, I felt the loss keenly. I still miss his gentle humor, and his sometimes less gentle reprimanding of the other guys when their jokes got too off-color. The crowds had felt a little safer when he was around. I once heard of death described with a metaphor of a beautiful garden. When we lose someone, it is like a rock falls into our garden, destroying the plants around it. Over time, flowers and vines grow around the rock, and the garden becomes beautiful again, though the rock is still there.

Rob made a number of handwritten posters, reminding volunteers to rinse out the mops or sort the recycling. Although I print most signs on the computer, opting for a more legible look, I preserved a few of Rob's notes in plastic covers, in part to keep him with us. Few people recognized his writing, but those notes were an anchor to me, a rock in our garden.

If I had known how much navigating grief—both my own and my hungry friends—would be part of my job description, I am not sure I would have taken that first summer job that set me on this path. Yet, I also suspect that no other path would have been as rich, or would have allowed me to befriend someone like Rob.

Helping people to navigate grief is generally seen as a counselor's or pastor's job, certainly not the role of the dietitian or program coordinator. I have felt gratitude, over and over, for my colleagues who can focus on people in crisis while I hold the logistical threads, yet I am learning to see the things someone like me can do to help people navigate the heartache and soul-ache that is so intermingled with bellyache. German has a term, *kummerspeck*, which loosely translates as "grief bacon." It refers to the emotional eating we do when we need solace. Unlike *comfort food*, *kummerspeck* is not associated with anything potentially healthy.

The way through grief includes acknowledging it, talking about it, and finding ways to take good care of each other and ourselves in the process. Just like the smell of bacon that lingers well after it was cooked, grief cannot be contained or ignored. We will cycle through feelings of denial, anger, and sadness, which can hit us at unexpected times, years after the loss. Grief is sometimes expressed as distaste for something served at a food program, though it takes a good deal of groundedness to interpret, "Your food/portion sizes/coffee are shit!" as "I am brokenhearted and I do not know how else to express it."

The day after Robin Williams died by suicide, I spent twenty minutes consoling Jerry, a distressed volunteer. I do not usually follow the lives of celebrities, but the actor's death was a shock, and it was covered widely in the media. Jerry saw himself as being connected to Williams (though neither their physical appearances nor senses of humor had ever struck me as even remotely similar), and he was shaken up by the death.

I usually embrace moments when people open up and relate on a deeper level. This morning, though, we were trying out a new style of serving our community lunch, and we still had a number of details to figure out. I felt a surge of annoyance with Mr. Williams for his inconsiderate timing, as I did not have the time to debrief his death or address the issues it was bringing up for Jerry. Celebrities really ought to consider the impact of their actions on people like me who are trying to put community development principles into practice and who may be in a critical stage of transition.

I had no idea about Robin Williams' struggles, and of course I do not want to make light of his despair. Thinking of the profound pain that he must have felt really saddens me. I grieve for the incomprehensible distress he, and others who come to the point of wanting to end their life, have felt. Sometimes, all we can do is return to ancient spiritual practices, set the table again, and again, and share our *kummerspeck*, lettuce and tomato sandwiches.

Fasting and Cleansing

"Can I be vegetarian for the next three weeks?" a client asked one day. The church he was attending while he was in a recovery program was encouraging its members to try the Daniel Fast, eating only water and vegetables, or only foods that come from seeds, according to one translation of the Old Testament passage in Daniel 1. He seemed so excited and hopeful about this fast, and about what he was being taught on how to spend the time on spiritual practices that he otherwise would have spent eating.

I get a lot of questions about fasting, cleansing and detoxing from people who are looking to cure an addiction, or who have realized that their attempts at self-medication were ultimately too costly, or have recognized that sobriety has a spiritual dimension. I respond to questions about fad detox diets with the idea that our bodies are detoxifying at that very moment, our kidneys and livers being pretty cool organs that chug away no matter what we are doing.

Intentional cleanses or detoxes can be beneficial, in large part because we cut out the ultra-processed, food-like snacks that our bodies are not really designed to process. Fasting, or deliberately abstaining from food, or just certain foods, may be necessary before some medical procedures, and certainly can have positive physical and emotional benefits. Many spiritual and philosophical traditions encourage fasting as a regular discipline, reminding us to be more intentional about actions that may have become automatic and thoughtless.

In response to an individual's questions on fasting or cleansing, we would address, if it had not been part of our earlier conversation, how hunger makes us irritated and distracted, and often leads us to make decisions we would not make when we eat well. Fasting should generally be attempted when one is in a relatively strong place, not during times of acute stress or early recovery.

If individuals are still intent on fasting or cleansing, we discuss how they could start with a simple fast instead of cutting out all food, trying to cut out sugar, caffeine, meat, or dairy foods. It is helpful to stay hydrated with unsweetened fluids, and be prepared for tiredness, mood swings, cravings, or headaches, especially if one's body is used to regular caffeine and sugar infusions. It may be easier to slowly decrease caffeine over a few weeks, rather than stop suddenly.

If fasting, make time for other types of self care, such as rest, journaling and exercise, and to have a plan to deal with difficult emotions that will likely surface. I encourage people to be gentle with themselves if they break the fast before they planned to. Recovery and wellness are a long, non-linear process. Nothing in nature blooms continuously, and neither will we.

When one returns to regular eating after any time of limited eating, it is best to start slowly, and to avoid eating until we feel overly full. Bodies will likely have lost water weight, which will come back quickly. It takes time for our appetite and digestive system to re-regulate, and it is common to feel some nausea, constipation, or other physical symptoms. Talk to a health care provider if the symptoms are distressing or last more than a few days.

If attempting a longer fast (more than a day or two), let someone else know what you are doing and how long you intend to fast. While fasting is meant to be a private discipline, the impact on vulnerable bodies can be significant, and it is a good safeguard to have someone else know what is happening.

After setting up what I could with the food services department for the three clients who were attempting the Daniel Fast, I was still uneasy about whether it was a good practice for them at that time. In the end, two seemed to do well with the exercise, but the third client relapsed and left the center before the end of the week.

I checked my go-to references for a handout on fasting and cleansing during early recovery, but could not find one, so I created one, pulling together what I knew about different aspects of both fasting and addiction. When I had a solid draft, I sent it to a few colleagues for vetting. One friend, after correcting some of the language that was too clinical, included in her message to me, "I stopped and thought about whether I had eaten appropriately today or whether I made any poor decisions related to hunger." Even when we earn a good salary, have a home, and know how to take care of ourselves well, we still need reminders of the connection between what we eat and how we cope.

I went for a walk the evening after I heard that the client who was doing the fast had relapsed, initially being hard on myself for not trusting my gut and intervening more. I walked along one of Vancouver's ocean paths, where the light was perfect and the temperature suited my mood, and my body responded with increasing energy. I fell into a rhythm of steps, partially noticing what and who was around me, but partially thinking how I would respond next time I faced a similar situation. Had anyone else stepped into a role that seemed simultaneously natural and far too large? Did anyone else find themselves in a community where they felt like they were both an insider and outsider?

Some days, when I walk, I hope I will meet someone—a friend, or acquaintance, or a stranger. That day, I hoped I would not, but I did see someone I knew from the food program circuit. We made eye contact, so I stopped to greet him. I did not know him well, but well enough to sit down next to him when he seemed keen to talk. I did not bring up my dietitian-failure-of-the-week, but as we talked about other things, I was reminded that the larger network of supportive programs in this city was ultimately doing good, and reminded that I should stay the course. My spiritual guides show up in unexpected places, but they do show up when I need them.

Chapter 5

Vulnerability and Resilience

Redemptive Pizza

Twice in one week, I sat with people I had just met, trying to figure out how to respond to their questions, conscious of the larger questions behind their spoken ones. I earnestly attempted to find something to say that would be comforting and honoring of the vulnerability they had just expressed, though that would have required the ability to freeze time and reflect for a while.

On a day that our community meal was not running, I was called out of a staff meeting and informed that someone had come by to ask a question about our dining room. I found Jon in the hallway, and introduced myself. He asked me if I knew a particular boy named Tim, about ten years old, with dark hair, who had been coming to the community dinners. I did know Tim. Only a few kids attended the meal, so those who did stood out. Plus, Tim's mom was vocal about her many diet restrictions, and we would try to find foods she could eat when she came. In response, she would nudge Tim to come find me after the meals to say thank you.

Jon told me that he was separated from Tim's mom, and she could get angry if he showed up where she was. He was concerned that she had some mental health challenges, and was self-medicating with illicit substances. Their son was on the autism spectrum, but the mom was unwilling to label the boy and get professional help. Tim had told his dad that he did not like coming to the community dinners, which is understandable, as they are not set up for kids, and they would be noisy and overstimulating for anyone whose brain processes information differently. Jon was concerned about what kind of setting his son was being exposed to, but knew he could not show up and see for himself. I attempted to describe the meal setting and the colorful characters who ate there.

We prioritized keeping the dining room a safe place, so would not invite people inside who seemed like they would be disruptive, but we intentionally hosted the meal for people who would not fit in elsewhere, so many of our guests could be unpredictable, or easily triggered into strong emotional responses and four-letter words. Fortunately, good food, learning names, and grace-beyond-measure ensured that, in all my years, I have only seen one cup of hot coffee thrown in the face of another.

"If you had kids, would you bring them here?" Jon asked. As I paused to think of how to answer that, he went on, "By not saying 'yes' right away, I know the answer to that." It is hard to answer questions about my own kidlessness. I tried, again, to explain how we do everything we can to keep the dining hall safe.

When children are in the room, it usually changes the dynamic for the better. A few weeks earlier, a man had expressed his frustration with the person sitting across from him with an angry string of curses. His voice had grown loud enough to attract my attention. "Watch your language, there is a kid here," I said, motioning to Tim, and trying to keep my voice quiet enough to entice the man to calm down enough to hear what I was saying. It worked. The man apologized and allowed me to escort him to another table, away from what had triggered his outburst. I opted against telling this story to Jon.

By this point, Jon and I were sitting outside on a bench near our garden beds, and Jon was telling me how helpless he felt about how his boy was being raised by an unstable mom and her string of questionable boyfriends. Jon was far away from his family, and was passing up good job offers in another city, since he could neither leave his son, nor move away with Tim. He teared up a few times, and I tried not to think of the lunch or to-do list I had intended for that hour.

"What is Tim's favorite food?" I eventually asked, maybe nudged by the One who answers prayers for wisdom. That question seemed to shift the dynamic of the conversation, and communicate that we cared enough about Tim to make the effort to serve what he liked to eat when he was in a difficult setting. Fortunately, Tim favors pizza and lemonade, and the community who come to the meals (and I) also enjoy them. Pizza, with dough from scratch, is one of my favorite things to make when I have company over for dinner, at least for my friends who still get to indulge in wheat and dairy.

We had started making pizza at this program a few months back, after watching a video about a $1 pizza joint where someone came in one day with $2, eating one slice of pizza, and telling the cashier to give away the other slice to someone who needed it. The store manager overheard the exchange and liked the idea. He put a pad of sticky notes next to the cash register and let customers know they could pre-buy a slice of pizza, write a note on the paper, and stick it to the wall. Others could come, take one of the notes, and pay with it. One shot in the video showed a whole wall covered with colorful notes, and a woman saying that, when she needed it, she got pizza with one of the notes. Now that she was in a more stable situation, she herself was putting a few notes up on the wall. We need to spread more stories about that kind of creative generosity. Even pizza can be resilience building.

Jon left shortly after that, but his story weighed on me all week and brought up questions about whom we are serving. Do we focus on the homeless people in the neighborhood—the individuals whom the program was initially designed for? Or do we focus on kids like Tim, whose parents are in the midst of a seemingly insurmountable rift, and who would rather eat pizza in a quiet room with their dad than with dozens of unfamiliar faces?

How do we love a boy from a broken home, with his own way of processing the world, when he is brought into a setting that is not designed for him? Can we do something to shift Tim's path, to lessen the potential of him waking up in the alley across the street fifteen years from now, aching and unrested, and staggering across the street for a free meal and hot shower? I do not know the answer to such questions, other than to continue to welcome Tim and his parents into our lives.

Awkward-Vulnerable

Twenty-six hours later, I experienced another awkward-vulnerable moment of human connection. I was in the detox unit at a treatment center a few blocks away, trying to be a good example of a dietitian for the student who was shadowing me for the day. Two of the people in the group were dozing, but three were engaged, which is a pretty good ratio for this setting.

Diane, a client at the center, had joined the conversation after I invited her to leave the desk where she had been coloring. I had seen Diane in the neighborhood many times over the years. She walked slightly bent over, and it always reminded me to square my shoulders and pay attention to my posture. Now, when she stood, she was almost bent at a right angle. It baffles me that we cannot help people like her straighten out her back and live more comfortably. And it amazes me how someone like her can still be so cheerful in the midst of detoxing for the tenth time. Or maybe twentieth time.

It would be more accurate to say that Diane joined the conversation after she showed me the intricate underwater scene she had been coloring, and how it looked totally different when she turned it upside-down and sideways. I did not see what fascinated her so much, but did allow for a little extra time for her to join our circle and get settled. The group conversation went pretty well, and I made the points that were important—eat every few hours, but not to the point of feeling stuffed, be especially intentional about personal hygiene and food safe practices while their bodies were getting strong again, and stay hydrated.

I sometimes made this last point with a tumbler of amber-colored detox tea that was always available at the center. "If your urine is this color, the things your body is trying to get rid of are too concentrated. Drink more fluids, and you will probably feel better."

There is not anything particularly magical about the combination of herbs in the detox tea, but more non-caffeinated, non-sugary fluids, plus slowing down enough to savor a hot drink, is good for anyone, whether or not a body is experiencing painful withdrawal symptoms. Pointing out the color of the tea is an effective object lesson, but I then feel funny about sipping it through the rest of the session.

Detox Tea:

10 grams Catnip Leaf & Flower

50 grams Chamomile Flower

10 grams Hops Flower

10 grams Lemon Grass

30 grams Peppermint

10 grams Skull Herb

10 grams Yarrow Flower

10 grams Yellow Dock Root

When dehydrated, we can feel any number of symptoms, including aching body, mental fog, leg cramps, constipation, and fatigue. Anyone in a stressed state can forget to listen to thirst signals and let him or herself get dehydrated. A shelter guest told me he had been feeling ill one day, and, as we chatted, it became evident that he had had very little to drink that day. I briefly reviewed the symptoms of dehydration as I poured him a glass of water, and to demonstrate that he was tracking with me, he said, "I get you. My pee could peel the chrome off a trailer hitch."

At one point, someone in the group asked, "What's a carbohydrate? Aren't those bad for us?" I explained the difference between carbs and protein (fats being too complex for the conversation at this point), and which healthier carbs were available for meals and snacks at the center. I hoped the student that was shadowing me was impressed with how I was handling the depth of questions, and how the group seemed to be responding to the information. When it felt like we had covered enough, knowing it was better to be short and sweet, I suggested we wrap up for the day.

As everyone was leaving the room, Carl, one of the group members who had dozed through the earlier part of the session but was now alert, asked, "Can I ask you something, kinda private?" I sat back down, and leaned toward him, nodding. The student and Diane followed suit.

"Uh, it's private," Carl repeated, glaring at Diane. She got the message, and hobbled out of the room. I was about to ask Carl if it was all right if the student stayed, but he did not seem to mind that she was there. He began what felt like a confession about some excessive steroid use, and then explained how his male bits were not working. He wondered what he should eat to . . . um . . . be okay again. I should be prepared for these kinds of questions by now, and have done some pre-reading on such subjects (we had not covered this in dietitian school).

"That's not fixable. You pretty much hooped yourself," was my first thought, but that would have been neither true, nor professional, nor good mentoring for the student, nor kind to Carl after what must have been a hard question to ask. I did not try to answer his question directly, but reiterated the idea that all our body processes are interconnected, including our brains, and as we get into better self-care rhythms, we feel better, and function better overall. That seemed to satisfy him. I hope it was the right answer.

Listening for Vulnerability

Around that time, not long after Thanksgiving, I was invited to become part of the team at a downtown church that had started to address how its food programs impacted the neighbourhood. The first meal I joined the team for was delightful. I got to peel a bowl of potatoes, gaining both a sense of accomplishment for having done something useful, and a sense of how this team worked as I watched who did what. Someone made me a name tag, and then pinned another on the volunteer I was working with, apologizing that she could not get it straight. "That's okay, neither am I," was his response, illuminating how accepting this group was.

As lunch was being served, I sat down with a cup of coffee at a table, and met Allan, who was diabetic and a regular at this place. He explained these three details as if he were telling me his first, middle, and last name. I asked Allan if he takes medication, in part making conversation, but in part the dietitian in me was curious how much he knew about blood sugar control. The small tower of cookies in front of him made me feel some concern for his health. Everyone else had finished and left the table, so I presumed that Allan planned to eat all the cookies he had scrounged after others left them behind.

"I don't believe in medication," he said, then added quickly, "or in counseling or psychedelic drugs or mental health groups or meditation or conservatives or gay marriage, I take walks and have my coffee and pray and have lunch here 'cuz if I don't do these things I feel like hell." Then he took a breath, and explained a few more of his health tricks, jumbled up with theology and political views, his thoughts racing faster than his tongue could form words. I gathered that this lunch was a regular part of his weekly routine, providing some cadence and connection in an otherwise chaotic existence.

"Wow. I have never seen him talk so much," one of the regular volunteers told me after Allan left. This group was on the verge of making some significant shifts towards more inclusive, dignified ways of serving, but at that point, there seemed to be a number of unwritten rules about the role of the church volunteers. If they would sit down to talk or eat, or if guests helped in any way, the volunteers were not doing their jobs well. All week, my mind ruminated over how difficult life must be for individuals like Allan, and how simply listening can amplify our acts of hospitality.

A few days later, I read an email that was sent to a group I am connected with, though I will not specify which, since the message made me cringe, rather than feel what the writer had intended. It was a thank you note for everyone who had participated in a Thanksgiving meal prepared for several hundred people, many of whom would have had multiple other similar meals on disposable dishes that week, giving dozens of volunteers the chance to do something, *to give back*, as we like to say.

> Greeted at the door with a smile, enjoying piano music as they waited, and being served with compassion and kindness, I could see each person's dignity being reaffirmed, and hope being restored as they were touched by real warmth and authentic community.

"No! No, no, no. Sure, there were smiles, nice music, and kindness. But we did not reaffirm dignity or restore hope, and it was not the guests waiting in the lineup in the rain who experienced warmth or community," I replied. Or at least I wanted to reply-all.

Another organization released a short video that told the story of their Thanksgiving dinner, thanked their volunteers and donors, and talked about the community they had built. It was a touching story, and it did convey the compassion at the heart of the effort, but one shot in the video saddened me. In this moment, a woman who, from her physical appearance, seems to have had a hard life, is sitting alone at a table, in a roomful of people, with a full plate of food in front of her. Her cup, cutlery, plate, and placemat are all disposable, although there is a beautiful bouquet of flowers on her table. Rather than eat her entrée, the more nourishing part of her meal, she is holding a smaller plate with pie, about to take a bite of that. Serving dessert at the same time as dinner would never be done at one of my family gatherings, or at any formal banquets for those with more means. And while we must respect each person's autonomy, it is also right to help those who know acute hunger to eat well, which should include not enticing people with sugar before they have had a chance to consume some more solid food.

I am confident the food at those dinners had been good. If you have ever cooked a turkey dinner for twenty people and have wondered how to scale that up thirty times, the secret is to pay extra for deboned turkeys (or pre-roast, carve, and freeze the birds the week before, if you have the personnel and freezer space). Make cranberry sauce and stuffing from scratch (day-old bread is a renewable resource in the food charity world), combine powdered gravy mix with some turkey pan drippings, and then settle for instant mashed potatoes. Few people will notice the potatoes, and it will save you much needed time and space. If you plan the feast for the week after Thanksgiving, you can probably get enough pumpkin pies donated, too.

Celebrations and feasts are essential for every community, and meals that remind us of the abundance of harvest seasons are worth doing. But when they become routine and too large for your dining table, they tend to make a good story, but do not ultimately address the vulnerability of those who have neither a dining room, nor the budget, to host a feast for their friends.

That angst inspired Planted, the community food network I work with, to host a workshop to discuss holiday meals. We were all beginning to plan our Christmas dinners, repeating the large meals we made for Thanksgiving. As food program coordinators, caring support staff, and volunteers, we want the holidays to be a meaningful time for our guests, especially those who see the programs as their extended family. Yet our holiday meals tend to leave us feeling more exhausted than festive. We needed to brainstorm ideas on how to navigate what can be a tough season for many.

The individuals who came to the workshop talked about how social gatherings do inspire camaraderie and celebration, and, hopefully, a sense of belonging. They are often like a homecoming—people who have moved on return to the programs they were part of for the bigger feasts. Holiday dinners can be a safe place to be for a few hours, especially for anyone who would otherwise be isolated, or who could not be at a shelter during daytime hours.

This is especially important around Thanksgiving, Christmas and New Year's.

We talked about how there is value in reconnecting with traditions such as festive foods, music, and gifts. Food prepared for holiday meals is often more abundant and better quality than weekly meals (more meat and real whipped cream). Celebration dinners can be a time for the greater community to give more, and thus become more aware of those in need.

The people at the workshop also expressed concerns about what typically happens at larger holiday feasts. We are sometimes given inappropriate gifts that are meant to be passed on to community members, gifts from people with good intentions, but who do not understand the community, or who have their own agenda. There is a lot of giving (time, food, items. . .) around Christmas, and ideally that would be more evenly spread through the whole year.

When we plan special meals for large crowds, we often create new challenges and experiences that are stressful for guests, volunteers, and cooks, including:

- Increased waste.
- Crowds that lead to congestion, which, intentionally or not, makes diners feel like they should rush through their meals.
- Parachute volunteers who take tasks from regular volunteers, leading them to feel misplaced.
- The meal itself is often too large, and people leave feeling unhealthily stuffed. (One year, I spent weeks advocating that a program not order their customary white buns for Thanksgiving dinner, as the potatoes, stuffing, and pie would cover the carb quotient. My eloquent stubbornness eventually won over tradition, and the money they usually spent on buns was diverted towards something more nourishing, a practice I hope the program has kept up.)
- Chefs with limited experience in quantity cooking may pre-cook food hours ahead of time, which can compromise

food safety (vulnerable people are more susceptible to food poisoning).

- Efficiency can get in the way of organic connection.
- Larger crowds can lead to more incidents, so we need to be especially proactive about fostering safe settings.
- More people can compromise the family feeling and hospitable rhythms established during other meals.
- Changes are hard—this community, like all of us, tends to value structure and predictability.
- It is usually cold and wet around Christmas, at least in Vancouver, and lineups are especially hard in winter weather.

Since we had a room full of logistics experts, we came up with a list of actionable wishes for the upcoming festive seasons. Holidays can be a time to make new, positive memories, which are vital for those trying to maintain sobriety. We would renew efforts to coordinate organizations in balancing holiday meals over the whole season, and encourage some groups to focus on especially vulnerable sub-populations. We talked about how it is important to take special diets and preferences into account, making vegetarian, gluten free, and softer options.

We talked about how it is important to honor other cultures. We cannot assume that everyone follows European traditions of turkey dinners, December 25, and Santa Claus. Many in our community observe Orthodox Christmas in January, Chinese New Year a few weeks later, Eid Al-Fitr and Eid Al-Adha, whenever they fall in the Islamic lunar calendar, or other cultural holy days.

The group expressed mixed feelings about gifts. I have been part of some beautiful exchanges, and I have seen moments that exemplify the *better to give than receive* idiom. When organizing gifts, we must consider how much individuals can carry, and limit low quality items, especially cheap gloves. Personalized gifts work for smaller programs, but are impossible for larger programs where we do not know who or how many people will come. Many people find personal messages meaningful, though we cannot expect that everyone will. Recipients often prefer gift cards, though they are generally better when a relationship with the individual exists, as such cards are impersonal, and might be traded for something else. Creative examples exist of ways to help our program participants give gifts to people whom they care about, such as a "free store" where people can "shop" for items, or cards, envelopes, and stamps (plus help looking up addresses) to send greetings.

As many holiday meals are hosted by churches, we also talked about the spiritual significance of the Advent season, and how we did not want to let materialism get in the way of the real Gift of Christmas. Many Christmas songs have beautiful words, and are meaningful (or at least nostalgic) for our community. Still, we need to tell both sides of the Christmas Story—the grace and the sorrow.

More emotion may be felt and expressed at Christmas. We see and feel a lot of nostalgia, generosity, and positive sentiments, and we often witness an accumulation of hard emotions this time of year. Many in our community are grieving. One church responds by hosting a Longest Night of the Year Service of Lament. Another hosts Blue Christmas Services.

A final realization that emerged from the group discussion was a reminder that the holidays are often a particularly busy and heavy season for chaplains, shelter staff and other supportive program coordinators. They, too, need more sustenance than usual. A card, a batch of cookies, or offering up a lakeside cabin for a weekend once the bustle is over helps to embrace the next season.

Just as there are many factors that make people vulnerable, there are many things that build up resilience. I appreciate how these terms, which are an increasing part of the vocabulary in support programs, capture the complex reasons for individual struggle, and point to the holistic efforts it will take to support individuals so they are at the table with us.

HALT

One of the concepts often used in recovery programs to teach basic self care and emotional intelligence is HALT, an acronym for hungry, angry, lonely, tired. When we get into any of these states, we make poorer decisions than we would when we are in a better frame—physically, socially, emotionally, mentally, and spiritually.

I had been discussing this idea with Eric, a dinner guest who had made some dumb-ass decisions in his life (his words, not mine). That, coupled with growing up in a system that was difficult to navigate and not being given the resources to do that well, landed him in jail and, after that, in one of my food programs. It seemed like he was getting the idea of how eating more consistently would help him think better, and face what he needed to do to get back on his feet. Next, I wanted to address the idea that, for holistic health, it takes more than just consuming calories that prevent hunger. The quality of the food we eat also impacts how we cope. Eric had subsisted on a diet of ultra-processed food, and did not seem ready to embrace whole foods. I do not imagine his time in shelters had helped him develop tastes for ancient grains and plant-based proteins.

I tried an analogy, comparing nutrients to money. I asked Eric, if I were to hire him to move my filing cabinet, a monstrosity that I had inherited from my predecessor, would he prefer I pay him $10 or $20?

"Of course, the twenty bucks," Eric replied, and went on, thinking out loud, about how he got the point I was making about how he should try better food, maybe a few more vegetables, a few less fast food meals. As tempted as I was, it was not the time to give him a list of healthy snacks, or quick-and-balanced breakfast ideas, or go into why we should pause before putting anything into our mouths in the spirit of gratitude and mindfulness. Anything Eric remembered of this discussion would come from his own reflections. And so I let him talk for a few minutes, encouraging his ideas. Then he got a pensive look on his face, realizing the fallacy in my metaphor, and said, "But for you, I would move the cabinet for free."

Trauma Informed

There is a growing understanding that it is pain and trauma that make people unable to cope, and force life to spiral to a place where free food programs and crowded shelters are their only option. That is a more helpful lens than seeing someone on the street as delinquent, lazy, or entitled, as some might do. Any of us could come apart if three devastating things happen to us in less than six months—loss of a significant relationship, an accident, loss of a job, an illness, loss of a home—and we did not have a significant support network to help us deal with the compounding crises.

When we are in a calm setting, we operate with the part of our brains that can be creative, multi-task (though not as well as we think we can), connect with others, and relate experiences to emotions and memories. When something stressful happens, say large flames suddenly consume a tree right outside a room where you are hosting a community meal, or someone yells accusingly that you are going to hell because you charge $1 for a lunch that used to be free (honestly, I could not make these examples up), we flip into our fight, flight, or freeze response. Adrenaline starts pumping through our bodies, and we are primed to react.

A trauma, even if it was a relatively mild event experienced as traumatic, can cause the brain to flip into that same triggered state. It is like an allergy, where a particular food activates an immune response. Individuals who struggle to calm themselves after being triggered are sometimes unable to work or maintain relationships, and are more than likely to end up at community meals. Hunger and poor self care also decrease resilience and cause the flip to be more readily triggered.

At one community meal, a street-involved woman we got to know became part of the core volunteer team. She had been a sporadic guest at this weekly meal, and had knocked one day on the door of the church that hosted the meal, though it was not a day that meals were being served. She and her boyfriend were experiencing desperate cravings for nicotine and pot, respectively, and asked the pastor for money to get them through the day.

Normally, it would be considered poor pastoring to give money to people in a state like that, but, as she tells it, the pastor reached for his wallet and handed over a $20 bill. The fact that he trusted her with the money led her to start hanging around the church. She eventually became a central part of the meal team, moved into a house set up for people in recovery from addictions, married someone she met there, and at our last point of contact, the couple had moved back east to work in another recovery program.

The other thing I remember distinctly about her is that if anyone around her hummed, she would have an immediate, terrified reaction, and run from the room. She eventually told us that she had been assaulted while her attacker hummed, and the sound brought back the trauma. It was through befriending her that I began to understand how deeply a traumatic experience can affects someone.

Remembering her story reminded me to check in with her. I looked her up online and sent her a note. She had recently posted a picture suggesting that when experiencing an anxiety attack, it is grounding to find five things you can see, four things you can touch, three things you can hear, two things you can smell, and one thing you can taste. Exercises like this can help one regain a sense of control over their surroundings and their feelings. Maybe that pastor who gave the $20 a decade earlier had a sense that the person who knocked on his door would eventually be on her feet, using a worldwide social networking program to show off pictures of her dogs, and sharing reminders with her vulnerable friends of how to recover from traumatic moments.

Psychological Food Aversions

In the food charity realm, I occasionally hear beggars-can't-be-choosers type sentiments, though I have only heard once of someone actually saying that to a meal patron in response to his inquiry about an alternate to the entrée being served. The well-meaning volunteer realized that she had chosen the wrong idiom while the words were leaving her mouth, and this is hopefully an urban legend, though I ought not judge, as I, too, have used culturally inappropriate phrases on occasion.

I have been oriented several times to new programs, and included in my instructions was an explicit request not to believe the clients, residents, or guests when they say they have food allergies, as that usually means they do not like a particular food, and want something special made for them. The person orienting me seemingly assumed that I agreed that the crowd at that particular program was full of people who were guilty of trying to cheat the system. While most food service operations are busy, and we cannot ask for too many special accommodations, a trauma-informed lens teaches us to look at requests for certain foods differently.

"Hey, do you remember me?" Terry asked me one day. "I was here a few months ago. I'm the one who doesn't eat eggs." I had a vague memory of his diet from his last visit to the program. Since I was on my way to the kitchen to give our cooking team a tally of what special diets we were going to accommodate for that particular meal, I sat down beside Terry to ask more. There were eggs in the cake we were planning to serve for dessert, so I inquired if that would cause him an issue, or if it was the texture or taste of eggs that he did not prefer.

It was fine if eggs were baked into food, Terry assured me, but if he saw eggs, especially scrambled eggs, he got nauseous. We were in a quiet corner, and Terry started to talk about his mom, who had been a crack addict when he was young. One day, in the midst of some chaos, she had forced Terry to eat a plate of scrambled eggs. He had tried to resist, not wanting the eggs, but she forced him to eat until he threw up, and then forced him to eat that. I do not think Terry, shaking with grief and shame as he talked, had shared this story with anyone before.

We as caregivers do not need to know stories like that to provide trauma-informed care. In fact, it is often better to not talk about such personal experiences if we are not trained to respond, and cannot hold space for the individual to adequately process the hard emotions connected with the difficult memory. We can, though, learn to watch for signs of anxiety when someone tells us they do not want a particular food, and resolve not to dismiss the person's request. There is always some alternate we can whip up.

Vicarious Trauma

"What doesn't kill you will give you trauma." I was driving and chatting with a dear friend who was visiting Vancouver, catching up on the past two years since we had seen each other, and this struck us as funny. "I couldn't make a joke like that with just anyone," I told Ahna, but she was someone who could see both the humor in my stories and appreciate their heaviness. To stay in this kind of work, one has to be able to hold that tension. Many of our friends and program participants live with a lot of pain.

A scary story unfolded during my early years in Vancouver. Women were going missing from the Downtown Eastside, and for far too long, not enough people took this seriously. A pig farmer named Robert Pickton was eventually convicted in 2007 of kidnapping and murdering many of the women. While I did not know any of the women who died at his farm, it is common for regular program participants to stop coming. We rarely know if this is a good sign, meaning that they have moved to a better place, or if it means trouble.

Several years after Pickton's trial was over, a police officer who had worked on the case was interviewed on CBC Radio. I remember her talking about some of the things the police force had done well, some mistakes they had made that they could only see in hindsight, and some of the problems in the police culture that prevented officers from acting on leads sooner. Given that many of the women who were reported missing were Indigenous and struggled with addictions, the case had not been given the focus that it likely would have if it been happening in another population. I cannot comprehend the horror that some of these women have faced, and what it will take to prevent anything like this from happening again.

I heard part of that interview both driving to work, and on my way home from an evening meeting, twelve hours later. Sometimes, God, or *Good Old Dad* (an acronym I heard this week by someone who was just getting to know his Higher Power), must lead us to hear something several times in short succession if we really need to learn it. I remember the officer saying that, knowing all she now knew, she would not have chosen to work this case and, although she recognized that her experience was much easier than those of the women who died at the Pickton farm, she still experienced some vicarious trauma. She said that she has to work hard to cope with this, but she is a better person for it.

I think about that idea when I feel overwhelmed with fatigue, grief, inadequacy, or experience moments of compassion fatigue or vicarious trauma. I cannot remember the police officer's name, but I can hear her voice, ". . . I am a better person for having been through this." That inspires me to keep at it, and to see my work both as a worthy way to invest my life and as a spiritual practice that connects to something larger than myself.

Part of nourishing the whole person—body and spirit—is building up individual and community dignity, and making space for the extraordinary impact it has on our lives. To understand dignity, our inherent value and worth as human beings, we may have to explore further how our programs and our stance can wear it down.

Chapter 6

Dignity

The Taste of Respectability

I HAVE ONLY DUMPSTER dived for food twice. The first time, I tagged along with some punk Québécois girls whom I met at a free meal. They had made a temporary home in a cheap hotel on the east side of Vancouver and were volunteering for one of the community programs I worked with. I had a car, and they had heard of some sweet spots on the west side of town, so we set out to find the fruitful dumpsters. I did not have the nerve that they did to sneak into loading docks behind grocery stores, but many dumpsters were more accessible. After an hour, my trunk was full of what seemed like very edible crackers (dented packaging), leafy greens (only slightly wilted), zucchinis (a few bumps), and pound cakes (nothing wrong with them that we could see).

I left most of the food with the francophones, as my goal had been more to educate myself than fill my kitchen, but they insisted that they had more than they could eat. I did not tell the people I was living with at the time where their dinner had come from, as I did not trust that they would enjoy it as much if I did (nor will I note now exactly what year that was—sorry, housemates).

The second time I fished my dinner from a dumpster was on one of the more creative dates I have had. It was a scavenger hunt that culminated with dinner at a park from things I had found, foraged, or otherwise acquired, as per the step-by-step instructions I was given. Few people would think up a date like that, and maybe even fewer would enjoy it, but if I was not smitten with the boy before then, I certainly was after that night. We were just playing, though. While we may not have had too much expendable cash, we could still afford to buy fresh food, and did not have to face what many in our city, and around the world, face daily.

Hungry people do some dangerous things. Recently, I met a friend for lunch at one of my favorite local cafés. There was a scruffy-looking guy with a glass of water in the corner, sitting quietly while his eyes darted around the busy tables. I watched him as he watched people leave. He would quickly grab the last few bites of sandwich on their plates before the bussers did. That place did make particularly good sandwiches, but one has to be pretty desperate before food that strangers have left half-eaten becomes appealing.

Moments like this help me see malnutrition differently than my nutrition textbooks define it. The guy at the café likely had low iron stores and some protein deficiency symptoms, but more clinically significant, he was deficient in income and justice, and had likely over-consumed addiction, pain, rejection, fatigue, and marginalization. It is not so easy to replenish those needs, especially with the typical food line.

Revolutionary Salad Bars

On a cloudy July morning, I made my way to one of the missions in Vancouver for breakfast and to meet Christine, a volunteer who had been with the organization for several years, who was now asking if something better could be done with the food served. Walking down the sidewalk towards the entrance of the dining hall, I stepped around a man shooting something into a vein in his left arm. We made eye contact, and there was no aggression in his expression. A bit of shame, a bit of apology, but mostly a welcome-to-my-neighborhood half-smile. I chided myself for walking by him, not stopping to help, though I did not know what I could do in the moment.

Instead, my contribution that day would be to set up a salad bar inside, so when he came in for lunch later in the day, he would be able to brighten up his plate with a few colorful fresh vegetables, some canned beans, and whatever else we found in the storeroom. Just as importantly, he would be able to serve himself. If my legacy is simply to introduce more salad bars, with some kind of plant-based protein in them, into downtown missions, that will be enough.

"Salads are not really popular here," Christine said, after I suggested it as a simple way to balance out their typical meals. "Do you find that at other programs? Many people don't have teeth. And people do want their familiar comfort foods."

I agreed with her, and then pointed out that fresh vegetables are rare in this neighborhood, but there are people who appreciate them. Even if only a handful of the guests opted for the salad bar, it was still worth setting it up. With toddlers, we sometimes have to introduce foods thirty times before they learn to like them, an approach that can work with adults, too, as we develop tastes for better food. If we set out leafy greens, cut-up vegetables, and chickpeas, lentils, or some other legume in the salad bar every day, eventually more people will start adding them to their plates.

"We could have a small salad bar," Christine conceded, thinking out loud, struggling to visualize how it would fit between the pasta and sandwiches they typically serve. "It would be tight, but we could fit another volunteer on the line to serve it."

"Not on the food line. What if we set it up at the end of the serving line, on the table where the tubs of bread are?" I suggested, walking over to the area.

"And let people just serve themselves?" Christine dismissed the idea as preposterous. There is something fun about radical new ideas, pushing boundaries—equal rights for people with different skin colors, women getting to vote, gender-neutral bathrooms (the hot topic in the news that week), and street-involved people enjoying a salad bar. I felt for a moment what must have motivated revolutionaries who changed the world so significantly that their recognizable images are now plastered on t-shirts around the globe. I only have influence in this small part of the world around me, so I will nudge what I can toward a better place. At least toward being a place I would want to eat.

I assured Christine it would work. Whatever food was set out would be composted at the end of the meal, not saved for tomorrow's soup. When she questioned what we would do about salad dressing, I said it was often served in plastic squeeze bottles. I shared a bit of wisdom I had heard somewhere, and adopted as my own philosophy: decide how much food you have to serve, share it open-handedly, and when it is gone, it is gone. Most guests will be respectful enough to ensure that the people behind them also get something. And if the bottle is only half full when it is set out, people tend to take less.

"But there are hoarders. Do you see people at other meals who bring containers and take everything they can? They will take all the food we set out." Christine continued to run through the protests that she knew the other volunteers would produce.

I assured her again that it would work, and that it was okay to communicate that when the food is all gone, that's it for the day. Plus, individuals with hunger-induced hoarding tendencies do not tend to stockpile raw vegetables. And, if the salad bar were at the end of the serving line, individuals would already have something on their plates, so the temptation to take too much would be less.

I explained how another site filled hotel pans with two inches of water, froze the pans, and then put the salad bar inserts in there. The ice lasts as long as the meal, keeping the items in it cool and crisp. The site did this for several years before finding a donor willing to pay for a permanent salad bar. Since that salad bar became a reality, I believe I can do anything—all it takes is three years of gentle, persistent requesting. It may have helped that the center's executive director loved onion rings, and I also approved a new deep fryer when the old one was no longer safe to use. Fish that gets donated to such programs tends to be less than fresh, and thus deep-frying makes it more palatable. I subtly worked the salad bar and onion rings into every conversation with my boss until she approved the purchase.

"We do have a big bag of dried cranberries. They could go into the salad bar, couldn't they?" Christine said, slowly coming around to the idea. We walked back to the storage area, and Christine told me about a friend of hers who came down to take some portraits of the participants in an art group at the mission, and then took some artistic photographs of the cans of food. Now it was my turn to have trouble visualizing how shelves of canned beans can look picturesque. We need artists in our lives to help us see the ordinary in creative new ways. I suggested we take a picture of our improvised salad bar, which might induce funders to help out, and persuade the we-have-not-done-that-before-thus-it-will-not-work volunteers to see the potential of color. We wandered through the storage shelves, an impressive collection, pointing out things that could go into the salad bar—beets, lentils, artichoke hearts, salmon, mandarin oranges, chickpeas. I resisted the urge to dust some of the cans and check expiry dates. I will try to do that on my next visit.

A few hours later, as I left the center, the man who had been sitting on the sidewalk as I arrived was still there, now with a small canvas, paintbrush, and set of paints. He was painting a bouquet of red roses, the brightest bit of color on the block. Before I retire, he will be inside washing dishes, maybe getting paid in cans of tuna, his art hanging on the walls, his name known by the others, his grandmother's salmon cakes recipe on the menu for lunch. Though it is perishable, too, that is what dignity tastes like.

Othering

As we explore how we share food, especially with those who do not earn enough to have a home and a stocked kitchen, or with those who experience some extraordinary brain functioning patterns, or with those who carry pain, we must be aware of the lens through which we see our dinner guests. It is all too tempting to commit "othering," or "otherizing," which labels someone as being outside our circle, too often belonging to a more undeserving tier.

When I started coordinating the Oasis Café, a weekly free meal in central Vancouver, the program had been going for at least a decade. It had a good momentum to it, but there were a few things that did not sit right with me. At that time, it was called Oasis, which was an apt name for what the founders of the program had intended to create, but over the years, the food line had become crowded and had settled into some chaotic rhythms. It would take us two years to brew up the café elements, and I am grateful to the team for their creativity and willingness to experiment.

The church building where the lunch is hosted has a large kitchen, a lounge on the west side, and a hall on the east side where tables are set up for the guests. The program had settled into a more-or-less efficient rhythm, where doors were opened two hours before lunch was served. Coffee was set up, and guests were invited to come into the oasis, out of the cold.

It was a good community space. The volunteer team buzzed around happily and busily in the background, making lunch, brewing coffee, and wiping up spills. Sometime, mid-morning, once the meal was well underway, one of the team would announce that it was coffee break time. Volunteers would fill ceramic mugs with coffee and real cream, and sit down in the lounge for a break. At the same time, the guests were in the hall on the other side of the kitchen, drinking their coffee out of Styrofoam cups. If they did not prefer it black, their only option was to whiten it with corn syrup solids and partially hydrogenated oils, more commonly known as non-dairy creamer.

With each passing week, I became more uncomfortable with the division. I do not think the volunteers were conscious of their *othering*, but the two-tiered coffee breaks had become part of the rhythm. I could not bring myself to use a disposable cup and powdered creamer, but I also could not sit in the lounge with the volunteers when I wanted coffee, separated from the people I was trying to understand.

I eventually decided that I could justify pouring coffee into a ceramic mug and carry that into the hall, even though the guests were drinking out of Styrofoam. I could not create more landfill when there were plenty of mugs in a rack on the other side of the wall from the stack of soon-to-be-garbage disposable cups. It had been my New Year's resolution a few years earlier to use fewer throwaway cups (this was when travel mugs were just starting to become common), and I was still committed to that decision. Although ceramic or glass dishes convey more hospitality and dignity than disposable ones, it did not feel like I was flaunting my privileged position by holding a mug.

Then there was the issue of what to put in my coffee. That year, my New Year's resolution had been to learn to like my coffee without sugar. Health was certainly part of my motivation, but I must admit that it was more about image. People who do not take sugar in their coffee have an air of betterness about them in my circles. Since then, my resolutions have become less specific. Two years ago, I resolved to turn 40 gracefully, and the year before that, inspired by my friend Lisl, I resolved simply that it would be a good year.

At that point, I had not yet learned to drink coffee black. I still do not prefer it straight up, but with all the time I spend at free food programs, I have learned to endure this when real dairy is not available.

My first week at that program, in an act of solidarity with my guests, I put the non-dairy creamer into my coffee and sat down to visit. I know some people do not mind the stuff, and a few even prefer it, or are so malnourished that any opportunity for sweet calories is appealing. More than once, I have approached a guest at community programs with a carafe of coffee, and the cup that the guest held out to me was already a third full of sugar and powdered creamer. The dietitian in me wrestles with what to do. Adding excessive amounts of seasoning or flavor enhancers is known as *condiment abuse*, and is common with anyone who experiences erratic or disordered eating patterns. It ruins the food and is a kind of self-harm. The complex reasons that drive someone to do it are not easily addressed in a drop-in program.

I got through a few sips of that coffee with non-dairy creamer, and then took my mug to the kitchen and poured its contents down the sink. The next few weeks, I would pour cream into my coffee in the kitchen and carry my mug into the hall before sitting down with guests, but this, still, did not feel right.

I resolved that, before the end of the year, I would change a few things. I knew that I needed to build trust and understand the political dynamics before I could suggest altering the routines of the faithful volunteers. I had just finished a degree in health-care leadership, and the theories we studied about organizational change and managing transitions were proving true.

The environmental concern seemed easier to address. I must credit the team because they were willing to wash extra dishes, and credit the church for buying enough ceramic mugs for all our guests to use. The volunteer team expressed legitimate concerns about people taking or breaking mugs, but within a few weeks they had settled into the rhythm of setting out and washing the mugs. A few might break or go missing most weeks, but replacing them was no more costly than buying the disposable cups.

The non-dairy creamer was harder to address. There was concern about storage, guests drinking whole glasses of milk, and cost, though we could buy a lot of milk for the same amount we spent on each 25-pound bag of whitener. I knew I could not change routines too quickly, but one week, the whitener was out of stock at the company we ordered supplies from. I could have gone to a grocery store, but I opted instead for a small stretch-of-the-truth and told the team that the whitener was used up, not available, and we had to try real milk that day. Despite their misgivings, the volunteers allowed me to serve it.

I promised that I would make it clear to our guests that the milk was for hot beverages, not for drinking on its own, though it soon became important to everyone that we offer a glass of milk to any kids who visit our program. When I made my usual welcome announcements to the guests, I mentioned the milk and asked everyone to use it for tea and coffee only, ensuring there was enough for everyone. The room exploded in applause, and one guest came up and hugged me. We did not go back to the powdered whitener.

What my hungry friends and I put in our coffee is a small detail when looking at our larger food systems and economic differences. I share this story as an example of how programs that exist to help those living in poverty can settle into practices that reinforce the differences between people, and as an example of what it takes to shift from a comfortable routine to a better practice. In Vancouver, most of us have strong feelings about our caffeine habits, and can empathize with the injustice of bad coffee.

I have addressed the use of powdered whitener in several food programs. Admittedly, there is some selfishness in prioritizing this, since it is easier to talk with guests and volunteers over a snack or drink, and I want real milk in my coffee, but it has become symbolic to me as one of the marks of hospitality. Nutritionally, a splash of milk may not make a big difference to someone with erratic food intake, but limiting the chemicals we feed people is always right. And offering the same things to our program guests as we consume ourselves is also significant in the move towards our higher common denominators—equality, dignity, and ceasing any othering.

Dignity & Employment

"Karen, I'd like to come back and be a volunteer again. Help you, you know," Kyle told me one morning. He was an exceptionally thin guy in his late forties, give or take ten years. Poverty can camouflage age. He was a friend of one of our regular volunteers, and had been a part of our team for a while, after which we hired him on to the Oasis Café's low barrier employment program, but somehow the process overwhelmed him, or other factors in his life defeated him, so he disappeared for a while. Eventually he came back as a dinner guest, sometimes friendly and charming, sometimes agitated and talking to people no one else could see.

Kyle had one good hand and one arm stub with something like fingers around where the elbow should be. When he first arrived, he told me he had experience washing dishes, and to my surprise, he could steadily plod through the ever-growing pile of baking trays and dirty plates. Never dismiss someone by his looks, his language, or his lack of a hand.

Years earlier, at a community kitchen, a guest showed up who had no real hands, just similar arm stubs and deformed fingers. I wanted him to feel like he was participating, so I set him up at a side table with one of my regular volunteers to make the cake that was going to be dessert that night. I figured he might at least be able to grasp the wooden spoon and give the cake batter a stir. I quietly suggested this to the volunteer, who I knew had the ability to engage easily with whomever walked through our doors, but who had less cooking experience than I gave him credit for. A cake should have been easy, with a clear recipe and all the ingredients pre-measured in little bowls. When I came back to check on them a few minutes later, the man with deformed arms was showing the volunteer how to crack open an egg.

The morning that Kyle wanted to volunteer, he was either a little buzzed or in a manic swing, as he talked more than usual. "You wouldn't have to pay me. I just want something to do. But if you pay me, I would send some money to those kids you see on TV, you know, in Africa, where you send in money every month to help them. I would like to help them." I was touched that Kyle would want to do this, suspicious that an addiction was trying to manipulate me into giving him money, disappointed in myself for being immediately suspicious, and frustrated that I could not help Kyle with either his desire to do something constructive for a few hours, or with his wish to support children even poorer than he was.

As Kyle looked at me expectantly, I remembered an idea cited in *Sweet Charity*, by Janet Poppendieck, about how reciprocity "is a fundamental organizing principle of human societies; both giving and repaying are demanded by social groups, and these obligations are maintained by sanctions including dishonor, guilt, and shame."[1] Just as I feel more at home when I can help my host with a meal I am about to receive, Kyle was wanting to participate in his community, but in that moment, I could not take him on.

We had a youth group visiting the city, doing *missions* for a week, and they needed some extra wrangling. My core team seemed to have lost their work ethic that morning, and the tables were a mess, the person assigned to bus them was nowhere to be found, and the cooks were behind schedule, having not quite figured out batch cooking. In addition, two pastors from nearby churches were visiting, having come to check out the set-up of our meals. The only thing that was going well was the mint-lime lassis that we had made with the abundance of fresh mint picked that morning from our garden. We had scrapped our other dessert idea since we had some plain yogurt to use up, and sugar and lime juice on hand. Blend all this together, add a little water if needed to get a pourable consistency, and it will make a simple, refreshing dessert for any hot day.

An hour later, everything and everyone was more settled. I saw Kyle sitting outside on the steps, where he was rolling something in a little square of tissue paper. Again, my first thought was not generous towards him, but more related to how I would make clear to him that his rolling a joint in front of pastors, innocent youth from a small town on Vancouver Island, and our vigilant neighbors would make me look like a poorer manager than I already was, and this was not the day for that.

I approached Kyle, considering what to say, and decided it was most likely tobacco he was rolling, not something illicit, and that it was not worth asking him to leave. He asked, again, if he could help me. I, again, told him we had all the help we needed. He accused me of not liking him. I tried to assure him that was not the case, and wondered what Jesus would say when accused in such a way. Our conversation was interrupted by a man who had just parked at the curb near the stairs where Kyle sat, and who began yelling angrily as he opened his car door.

1. Poppendieck, Janet. *Sweet Charity?*, 251.

Two men got out of the car parked in front of him. They had a different skin color than the first guy, and had just come from lunch at our community café. My guests had thrown some beer cans out of their car onto the sidewalk, and the man who had parked behind them was curtly suggesting that littering was disrespectful to the neighborhood. It surprised me that a carful of men like that would drive to our lunch. If they could afford a vehicle, insurance, fuel, and beer, they were not the people I was cooking for. But there are deeper, systemic issues, I know.

So, while trying to assure Kyle that I did not have a grudge against him, I watched the fight about to explode. "You want a piece of me?!?!" yelled the driver-who-did-not-recycle, walking toward the other man. My nervousness grew as I watched this exchange, though I was amused that people actually use that phrase.

"Is everything okay?" I asked, a little lamely, conscious that I was not carrying my phone to call for support, or at least pretend to call, which can be equally effective. Realizing that they were being watched was enough to dispel the tension, and the men got back into their cars and drove away in different directions.

"Kyle, would you go pick up those beer cans?" I was just as relieved to have a job to give him as I was for not having to call 9-1-1, sweep up broken glass, fill out an incident report, explain to the visiting volunteers that we really are a safe place almost all the time, and revisit our Good Neighbor Agreement, having reminded the wary people who live in the nearby apartment buildings that our meals do attract some shady characters. Finally, I could go inside and find something to eat before all the food was given away, and Kyle could earn a dollar with the cans.

Another day, I walked into the dining room at the same program, and heard, "F-this. F-you. F-him! F-God! F-ev-e-ry-one!!" Kyle's volume was growing with his agitation. Mario, who had the patience and life experience needed in this setting, and who had visited the community meal one day and before long was helping to run it, was gently ushering Kyle outside. It seemed like a change of connection might help, so I walked over to Kyle and attempted to engage him. It was almost like he was rapping a rhythmic expression of everything that was messed up in his world. We got him outside, and he calmed a little. I asked him how his day was going. He responded with, "Wouldn't you, if someone said something like that to you, tell them to F-off?" I did not know what had triggered him, so I tried to draw the story out, and reassure him that it was our intent to make the dining room a safe place, but everyone had to help keep it safe. Kyle did not seem to pick up on the message that I was including him and his language.

"If someone treats you like that, you tell them to F-off. You can't just be pushed over," Kyle explained again.

"Actually, I would just walk away. Talking back usually makes things worse," I countered.

"Yeah, you're smart like that. I'm not smart sometimes. I just wanted to tell him 'F-you.' That would be the smart thing." Kyle was calmer now, but still not relaxed enough to head back inside.

"Kyle, would you sweep up these leaves here?" A chore would probably do more to calm him at that moment than any more dialogue. He agreed, and I went inside to find the broom and an extra dessert. There is a time and place for using sweet treats to encourage responsible behavior, and this seemed like one of those.

Never Wet Your Boss

I once read a poem about different levels of charity, the lowest being that the recipient knows who the giver is; the highest, that the recipient gets to earn their sustenance. I did not understand it at the time, but increasingly I do. When I started at the Oasis Café, the community volunteers who themselves lived on limited or no income were given $10 or $25 grocery store gift cards. These gift cards engendered a stable volunteer team, and I had a core of about fifteen people from the community who were at the meals almost every week. They knew each other and the tasks that needed doing, which made my job infinitely easier, though I disliked the transactional way I had to grab a stack of these gift cards from a locked cabinet in a locked office, note what I had taken in a benevolence log book, pull out our list of names at the end of every evening, dole out the cards, and check off who got what.

Some people would graciously receive the cards every time, and others would say something like, "Hey, Karen, where's the plastic?" then disappear as soon as they had it. Others would get upset, saying, "What?!? Are you paying me $2 an hour?" I would explain, again, that I was not paying them. I was thanking them for volunteering, while trying not to question their sense of entitlement or judgment, as they had just enjoyed a free meal. The gift cards were for a chain of stores which we thought did not sell cigarettes, but our enterprising crew had found the one store in this chain, a fifteen-minute bus ride plus twenty-minute walk away, that did sell them.

One day, Chad, one of our regular community cook volunteers, arrived noticeably intoxicated. There had been a hockey game, and being an avid fan, somehow owning two oversized jerseys, Chad had been enjoying the game and a bit of barley soup at a nearby pub (his preferred euphemism for beer). I had borrowed one of Chad's jerseys when I had been given tickets to a Vancouver Canucks game some months earlier and, since then, he had assumed I loved hockey much more than I did, and kept me informed of the season's stats and player gossip.

"If you are going to drink, you can come as a guest to eat, but not to volunteer," I explained to Chad, not sure how much of our conversation he would comprehend. He had started to act as if the program could not run without him. Chad was the kind of guy who noticed when some food scraps had fallen on the floor, and would scoop them up and toss them in the compost bin while he was engaged in other tasks. This level of conscientiousness was rare in our community, and I initially appreciated it, but his attitude was becoming a hindrance.

"So I need to treat this like a job?" Chad asked in response. I cannot call that my "a-ha moment," because it usually takes me time to reflect on things and realize their meaning, but that comment did change how I viewed and talked about volunteer roles, and was one of the factors that led us to create the low-barrier employment pieces of the Oasis Café. I realized how much my work gives me identity, security, affirmation, and an invaluable weekly rhythm, and how much more people without the ability to work need similar anchors.

I have long been intrigued with the people who show up at these free community meals as guests, and who take the initiative to help out, or who have natural leadership abilities, or who are asked to help when extra hands are needed and then quickly become part of the core team. The programs that can allow for this are the ones that have not run out of energy. These guys know the community far better than I, or anyone who has never lived on the street can know it, and although their methods are often gruff, their involvement is the real fruit of the programs.

After that conversation with Chad, I began to talk differently about the roles our volunteers played, saying things like, "It is okay to take a day off, in fact we encourage it, but please just let us know." I did not encourage anyone to call me "boss," but I tried to live up to the title when people used it. Like the day Sue was washing dishes and she asked me to step away from the counter so she could spray it down without splashing me. "Never wet your boss," I heard her earnestly explain to the new volunteer she was training.

Chapter 7

Healing Relationships

Redemptive Narratives

I ATE LUNCH WITH Mak at a community dinner one day. He had wandered up to me part-way through our meal service and said he had a few questions. I figured he was going to ask for socks, or explain his perspective on why it was good or bad that we had introduced a donation for the meal, and I was tempted to pass him on to someone else. We had only one new volunteer that day and he had found his niche as our bus person. Everything else was running smoothly, so I allowed myself a moment to pour a cup of tea, and then I walked over to the table where Mak was sitting alone. He was an older Indigenous man with a long braid and haggard face. I had seen him before at the meals, but had not had a conversation with him.

"I need to see a counselor," said Mak, in response to my greeting as I sat down. "All my relationships are not working."

"That's a big step. Good for you," I responded, surprised at his admission, my mind running through options to connect with a counselor, but sensing that it was not yet time to offer help. His story poured out as we ate our dinner of sesame chicken, quinoa pilaf, kale salad, and banana muffins, a fusion meal from the ingredients that had been on sale, donated or were left in our pantry. Mak told me about hard experiences in a residential school, and how he violently lost a number of people in his life whom he had loved. He wore a heavy coat of trauma and grief, and could scrunch up his eyes in a way that was almost theatrical, yet I could see pain in his face that made my heart ache. There was something else that sat heavily with me, but I could not articulate it until I was reflecting on our conversation later that day. There was no hint of communion or agency in any of Mak's stories. No narrative of something redemptive unfolding from the hard things he had experienced.

I tried to listen to Mak's story, to affirm the sorrow, to connect, to empathize, to help him find words for what he was feeling. But as he scrunched his eyes for the fifth time, at least, I thought about how his story was only one of lack.

"Do you have any good memories from when you were a kid?" I asked, trying to turn our conversation. He could not think of one.

"Do you know anyone in your family who is doing good things?" I tried again, still hoping to brighten him up, as I realized in a deeper way how historical trauma continues to manifest. Mak could not say one positive thing about his people. He continued his tale of woe by pointing out his eyes, which were the same color as mine. Our driver's licenses would say plain old blue, but I like to think of them as hazy gray. Mak had inherited his eye color from a Norwegian grandmother somewhere down his line. He told me this as a matter of shame—he was neither Cree nor Caucasian, so both tribes had rejected him.

"Do you know much about her?" I asked, my imagination intrigued by the woman who had braved the New World, left her people and all that was familiar, learned the Cree language and customs, fallen in love with Mak's grandfather despite the warnings from both families, and embraced her new life. The real story could have been more violent and tragic, but it could have included Mak sitting on her lap as a young boy, gazing into a face that was not like his, but with eyes that were.

Later that night, I met with some friends for dinner. Our conversation got around to compassion. My friend had recently been at a retreat with a Jesuit priest who had found his niche working with busy executives looking for spiritual grounding. During the retreat, they had explored the phenomenon of how when we see something familiar—a face, a place, a food—we have a positive physical reaction, with hormones, neurotransmitters, and other subconscious body processes evoking feelings of love and compassion. When we see something foreign, such as a face from another culture, or when we find ourselves in an unfamiliar setting, especially something that reminds us of something hard, we have an immediate and often unrecognized stress reaction. Our bodies are poised to reject *The Other*, but we can change that. We can intentionally wire our brains to learn to accept different things as something that is part of our tribe, and not a threat to us. We can convert prejudice into care if we think and act deliberately.

Mak and I were different on many levels, and maybe my initial hesitation to converse with him had been subconscious othering. But as I sat with him, I could feel compassion—we both needed lunch, companionship, healing relationships, and new perspectives. And our matching gray eyes made us kin, too.

Mennonites joke (though it is not really a joke) that when we meet each other, we spend the first moment with introductions, then the next few minutes figuring out how we are related. It is anchoring to know that the person beside you, who was a stranger a moment ago, is actually a third cousin, or the niece of our high school English teacher, or our grandparents' neighbor. My roots are not Norwegian, but they are Eastern European. Somewhere down the line, Mak and I could have inherited some of the same genes.

Talking about the lessons learned from the Jesuits led our group conversation to the story of the Good Samaritan, who found a beaten man from another culture lying at the side of the road. The Samaritan poured wine and olive oil on the man's wounds, took him to an inn, and paid for the innkeeper to tend to him until he was well. I had known this story from childhood, though

I had not remembered that the Samaritan had poured wine on the guy that was hurt. That detail had been omitted in my Mennonite Sunday school classes.

I wonder if, a year or two after he had healed enough to leave the inn, the man ever sat at a community meal or a pub, or whatever equivalent they had in his day (though I do know the story is a parable), and recounted his near-death experience. If he had, would he have told the story of the priest and temple assistant who walked past and ignored him, or would he have told the story of the foreigner who had helped? Was Mak sitting in a pub, telling his buddies about a pale-faced girl who had not listened at all to him, who did not understand his pain? Or was he telling a new story, one where he could remember something redemptive? Or had he completely forgotten our conversation, not continued to wrestle with it as I was doing?

Mother Teresa of Calcutta said, "Lord, when I am hungry, give me someone who stretches out their hand to me; when I am thirsty, give me someone who needs a drink . . . when I feel abandoned, find me someone to love."[1] When we are in a difficult place, reaching out to someone in an even more difficult place can turn our perspective, help us realize that we do have something to give, and in sharing what we have, receive something back. This is what I hoped for Mak, though I realized that his world and mine were so far apart.

It's the Systems, not the People

I pulled my compost bucket out of my freezer one Friday morning to toss in half a BBQ pork bun, leftover from a meeting I had attended with a group planning to show a documentary on food waste. I had promised not to let the bun go to waste, and ate half of it on my way to my next gathering, but then forgot it in my bag until the next day. What I saw in my compost bucket that morning dismayed me—this was during a season of living alone, not in a

1. Pious Society of St. Paul. *Blessed Mother Teresa*, 5.

shared home, and there was only one apple core and a pile of tea leaves in my compost. A whole week had passed since I last emptied the bucket, and I had not been home enough to make a meal for anyone or generate anything compostable.

My empty compost bucket indicated a rich and full life. I had eaten with my extended family on Sunday, and then at work or some other community event each lunch and dinner through the week. One evening, I had attended a dinner called Re-Plated, a multi-course tasting menu all consisting of food rescued from the landfill, served on platters made of refurbished scraps of wood from local construction sites. The dinner was organized by my friend Elaine, who finds creative ways to show how to reduce the amount of food we waste, both as individuals and as organizations. There has been a significant shift toward acceptance of *reclaimed* food in the past few years, but we still need people like Elaine to nudge us into better understandings of our food systems, and understand that food waste is not the solution to hunger and food insecurity.

As I reflected on my week, I felt grateful for the people and events I had connected with, but one interaction felt especially heavy. There is a man I will call Neil, whom I have been meeting at supportive programs in Vancouver for almost twenty years. Though he is Caucasian, he usually pulls chopsticks out of his pockets to eat at community dinners. Neil could only be described as gentlemanly, and he often makes the effort to thank me for the meals he attends, gently reminding me that he does not prefer beef, when that is on our menu, and occasionally sharing with me his working theories on government control or the commoditization of charity. One day he explained to me his suspicion that our national leadership was trying to eradicate broccoli from our landscape. Neil asked that I commit to work against this, should I ever see evidence of the villainous scheme. I assured him I would do my best, and then intentionally added more broccoli to the meals at the program where I most often met him those days.

Neil, who is probably in his late fifties, is currently living outside, though he has been inside for some of the past decade.

He does not like to be called *homeless*. He prefers the title of *landless peasant*. Over the past few weeks, I had noticed his hands become increasingly red and swollen. This week, the cracks on his skin looked excruciating. One hand was so raw that he could not put it in his pocket to get out the medicine he had just picked up. He asked me to check the pockets of his heavy winter coat. It is a strangely intimate thing to fish though the pockets of a jacket that someone else is wearing.

One of our volunteers took Neil to a shelter after dinner, unfortunately arriving too late, and he did not get a bed. Instead, Neil hopped on a bus and returned to the church just as I was leaving for the night. I had gone back to the room where we serve the dinner to ensure the lights were out and no one had fallen asleep in the men's shower, as had happened recently, understandably startling our janitor as he locked up for the night. It was 9:30 pm, pouring rain, and I was ready to head home. Just as I was about to switch off the light, I saw Neil's face in the window. Reluctantly, almost wishing I had not come down this way, and then scolding myself for such a thought, I opened the door and invited him inside. It is not the people who wear you out. It is the systems that are so hard to navigate.

"Do you think the Powers That Be would mind if I slept under the awning here tonight?" Neil asked, civilly. I told him that was not an option, but I gave him a blanket wrapped in a large plastic bag, a meager offering for a harsh night.

The next morning, Neil was back. We invited him in early as we set up for lunch. Neil had stayed in the parkade across the street until about 2:00 am, then had left because a large rat had run too near for his comfort. He spent the rest of the night tucked into an alcove of the church. He returned the blanket, and graciously accepted coffee and a slice of bread and peanut butter, which we kept on hand for our volunteers who would show up without having eaten breakfast. Cathy, a nurse who had moved to Vancouver from Germany and had not yet sorted out her credentials to work here, sat with Neil and helped apply the medicated cream he had with him.

At the end of a recent community lunch, Cathy mused that she was coming to see that meals are about so much more than food, and that she wished she could share that with our larger community. I wish I had a photo of the two of them sitting together as tables were set up around them. So many parts of our social support system are challenging to navigate, but there enough beautiful moments to inspire us to keep addressing the broken bits.

It Takes a Village

One early spring evening I found myself crouching in the rain, heavy rain, even for Vancouver. Next to me sat Meg, a regular volunteer at the community dinner, who had been asked to be away for a while after threatening another volunteer the previous week. The day leading up to that uttered threat had gone relatively well. We had made pumpkin soup and chocolate zucchini muffins (it was the time of year for the squash family), the dining room setup was completed on time, guests had arrived, and lunch service was underway. Then a volunteer, decidedly hungry, requested the person standing in front of her to move out of the way so she could find her server and get lunch. The problem, though, was that she did not use her friendly voice, and the person she tried to shoo away was her server, who did not respond well to the request or the way it had been delivered. I had stepped out of the dining room for three minutes, and when I came back, the two individuals, plus two more, were standing in a tight circle, loudly and simultaneously explaining their points of view.

In the previous hour, I had observed both of these volunteers engaged in thorny interactions with other individuals. Neither had seemed harsh enough to address, but both were enough to push someone with low resilience close to their tipping point.

Community meals may not be *real* restaurants, but we aim for some semblance of a fine dining establishment, trying to convey the dignity and welcome that anyone would feel when they go out to eat—greeted by a maître d', offered bread and a drink, and then asked what one would like to eat based on choices from the daily fresh sheet. Sometimes I feel hopeful about getting close to this ideal, and then sometimes my server, chatting with me during a slow moment, leans over, picks up an empty glass from my table, and pours himself a cup of water from the jug in front of me.

Another day, I had just reminded everyone to be sure they knew the ingredients in the dishes we were serving, especially since we were adding nuts to our spinach salad. One of my servers looked at the menu and said, "Borscht?!? What the hell is that?"

"We need to watch our language here," I tried to say playfully, teasing her, but also serious that I expected fewer four-letter words, and I expected her to be familiar with the delicious cabbage and beet soup that is the backbone of Mennonite cuisine.

"Yeah, or we'll have to take you out back and shoot you," said Ryan, another volunteer, joining the banter.

"Maybe we'll just wash her mouth out with soap," I said, still teasing, but also suggesting a less corporal punishment.

"Probably better," Ryan conceded. "I was a handful as a kid. From my experience, Ivory tastes the best."

So, imagine being at a restaurant, and seeing two waiters, the maître d' and another individual in the restaurant uniform, in a heated argument in the corner of the room. Rightly or wrongly, I marched up and hissed, "Not in front of the guests. Let's move this into the hallway." To me, this was a rational, compassionate, timely, simple solution. In a calmer setting, we could talk out the conflict while not scaring away our guests.

In the midst of conflict, the two individuals heard my suggestion differently. One heard something like, "I am asking you to do something you are physically not capable of doing right now."

The other heard, "You are being punished for this fight, and the other person, the one who hurt you in the first place, is getting off without consequences."

I did allow the one person to sit down, and did get Meg into the hallway, but the attempt to deescalate and bring back some loving feelings failed. She slipped around me to confront the other individual again, and this time a threat slipped out of her mouth:

"I am going to punch you in the face!" (Note: a few choice words deleted here.)

All this bubbled up more than it should have, and my colleague decided that Meg had to be away for a few weeks. Although we do take threats of violence seriously, I did not feel like it was the right response, but sometimes unity with one's colleague has to be prioritized.

Meg returned the following week, though she would not come inside. My colleague had tried to connect with her after the incident, but that had not gone well. Meg still felt like she was being unfairly blamed for the conflict, and her defiance had grown. I can only imagine what triggers from Meg's past hurts were set off. She had been asked to stay away, and when I reminded her of this, she countered by saying that she was there to say goodbye to her *friends* (her intonation made it clear that I was not currently part of that group), and she had every right to be on the property, though she had no intention of coming inside to help, or to eat. My colleague was dealing with the other person who had been involved in the conflict, which is how I ended up crouching next to Meg.

I had a good relationship with Meg, but I did not know if, still sore from the previous week's interaction, she would lash out in anger. As I tried to think of words that would communicate an apology plus loving boundaries, I sank down on another step, a few feet away. Before I could say anything, Meg looked down at me, took a moment to focus and realize who I was, and then said, "I just smoked something." She was completely stoned.

I felt momentary relief, knowing she was not going to start yelling, but then wondered if this could get even more complicated. We were meant to be serving dinner to the crowd inside in a few minutes, and I needed to be in there ensuring the last details were coming together. I managed to walk Meg across the alley and settle her onto a doorstep under an awning. With all her defiance gone, I could sense the hurt she must be feeling, and sadness over not being welcomed inside with her tribe.

A few years before this moment, several of the church's vocal neighbors had expressed their discomfort with our program and the kind of people we were attracting to the area. They made a formal complaint to city officials, who responded by ordering the church to apply for a social services permit. The church pushed back, arguing that part of our core mandate is compassion for the poor, and we should not have to obtain an extra permit to do so. It took several rounds of discussions, but the city council eventually decided that provision of services to marginalized people is the essence of the church, and thus no special permit was needed to run a community program.

In response, the church leadership had created a Good Neighbor Agreement, detailing the times that meals would be served and the precautions they would take to ensure the area was well cared for. Leaving someone in Meg's state on a neighbor's doorstep could be seen as violating our agreement. It had been several years since anyone had made reference to the agreement, and I did not want to remind any of our neighbors why it had been created in the first place.

I ran inside to check on dinner, then back out to Meg with a snack. She had a few bites, then pulled a $50 bill out of her purse and asked me to call her a cab. I knew she had an apartment in a social housing unit on the other side of town, and the cab fare would take most of her spending money for the month. I ran inside to check on the meal's progress, gave the okay to start serving, grabbed my keys and another volunteer, and got Meg into my car. Fortunately, she was alert enough to point out which building was hers, and we got her inside, where the building staff took over.

I met with Meg for coffee a few days later, still unsure whether she would be angry or receptive. My colleague had asked me to develop a return-to-work plan, which would include Meg apologizing to the person she threatened and to my colleague for some harsh things she had said. I considered how to address this, committed to ensuring that Meg also felt cared for and validated, and would receive an apology for what had hurt her. As we chatted, I decided we needed to build our relationship before I was in a place to ask anything of her.

Meg told me about her initial connection to a Christian church, when a friend had invited her to a Mennonite church in South Vancouver for a meal. Meg had returned for a service, and eventually been invited to have tea with one of the staff. The pastor, Ingrid, had made space to listen to the story of how Meg had fled her home in the Middle East, arrived in Canada with a young son, and struggled to raise him. As her story wrapped up, Ingrid had simply said, "I am so sorry. That must have been hard." Meg told me it was her empathy, and the fact that the pastor had not tried to give her advice, that made Meg want to become part of the church community.

Meg has visited the community lunch where I met her once or twice since that day, and we manage to connect occasionally, but she has not chosen to be part of our group again. I hope my relationship with her is not over, though there does need to be some healing, and I do not know how best to approach that. No multivitamin will correct these relational deficiencies. I can only trust someone else in this big village is walking with Meg now.

Healing our Relationship with the Earth

In 2010, Vancouver started working towards its stated goal of becoming the greenest city in the world, cutting in half the waste we generate by 2020, and moving toward zero waste by 2040. As we got closer to the 2020 deadline, city officials gathered together people who worked in charitable food programs, asking for feedback on the proposed next step—banning non-compostable single-use items like coffee cups, straws, take-out containers, and plastic bags. Knowing biodegradable items cost at least three times more than cheap materials such as Styrofoam, the people assigned to explore the ban wanted to know how this would impact charitable food programs, and how they could support the transition.

Vancouver had implemented a ban a few years earlier on food scraps and other renewable materials going in the garbage, and this significantly reduced the volume of what we send to the landfill. Charitable food programs now get more undesirable food donated than we used to, with businesses passing it along rather than paying to compost it, but the problem is not as bad as we expected when the food scrap ban was first introduced. We talk about how *free food is not really free*, as there is a cost to sorting and composting what we will not serve, though most organizations have set up workable systems to deal with inedible food.

In that meeting, city staff explained that, on our journey toward reducing waste, we had picked most of the low-hanging fruit, and now it was time to tackle harder issues. Vancouverites were throwing over two million cups in the trash each week. We pay $2.5 million a year for waste collection from our public garbage bins on streets, parks and green spaces, much of which is disposable food and beverage containers. While no one dares suggest we give up our coffee habit, there are ways we can make it less destructive. Most of us do not really think through what happens after we consume our caffeinated treats. Are cups recyclable? Compostable? What about the lids? Are we supposed to rinse the cup before we throw it in the bin? Are coffee grounds composted? What is done with the packaging for the coffee, cups, milk, sugar, and any other add-in's? What about the coffee growers—is our consumption leading to their flourishing? That last question is particularly important, but one to explore in another book.

The project team had met with manufacturers, business owners, lawyers, and others who are involved with making, buying, and selling food packaging, or developing laws around it. The team had researched what other cities around the world are doing, and had some innovative ideas to present, such as cup exchange programs, new biodegradable packaging materials, and public dishwashers.

Reducing waste is a strong value for me, as well as for many in this city—and I must give credit to my hard-working colleagues and volunteer teams for the extra effort they put into rinsing, reusing, recycling, and composting. At the end of a long shift, it is hard to still have the will to sort boxes, plastic wrap, and food scraps into the appropriate bins. Isaac, a volunteer chef who has devoted countless hours to local food programs, exemplifies the amazing people who help feed this city. As we are finally putting away the last clean pot and draining the dishwasher at the end of any given dinner, we will sometimes find a bucket with food scraps that no one took out. I can guiltlessly suggest we leave it until the next day, but Isaac will usually grab it and run it to the receptacle outside, saying, "Don't be that guy who leaves it for someone else." We are thankful in the morning, as it is so much easier to start the next meal with a pristine kitchen. When I lack motivation for clean-up tasks, I hear Isaac's voice in my head saying, "Don't be that guy, Karen."

After an hour of dialogue with city staff about how charitable food programs are doing what they can to reduce waste in their operations, someone voiced the idea that this discussion has to go along with a poverty reduction strategy. The rest of the group agreed, immediately adding suggestions. One thing I love about working in Vancouver is that there is always someone who sees the bigger picture, and will advocate for those in poverty. Food programs are important, but hunger will only cease to be a challenge when people have an income adequate enough to maintain a home and buy the groceries they need to feel healthy and secure.

Homelessness is a high-waste state to live in, with the programs we have set up to support higher risk individuals often requiring more single-use items. Without a home, one cannot keep a kettle and mug, or make coffee or tea in the morning. I can hardly imagine facing the world without some quiet time to wake up, think about my day, and savor the steaming cup of tea I just made. There is an encouraging *Housing First* movement emerging, based on the idea that most people will stabilize themselves once they have a secure place to live. We need to start there, not expect everyone to work their way through a rough shelter system or sobriety program before they are allowed keys to their own sanctuary.

Until all our neighbors have homes, there is still a place for emergency food assistance. It does not have to involve single-use containers, but it often does. Many organizations are taking good steps towards prioritizing hospitality and sit-down meals with real dishes, but there are times when an individual is too agitated to be invited inside a community space, or when individuals recognize they are not in a state where they can sit with other people, and packing up food to go is the best option. I used to be stricter about not allowing my food programs to become take-out joints, but as I journeyed with friends with concussions, I relaxed my stance, recognizing just how overstimulating a busy dining hall can be. I am reluctant to spend my food budget on take-out containers, so I compromise by encouraging people to collect plastic food containers that we can sanitize and reuse.

It is an art and science in knowing (guessing) how much food to prepare for community meals. We want to have enough for everyone, but not so much that we end up having to figure out what to do with a lot of leftovers. On slower (rainy or post-welfare) days, we sometimes have half-full pots of stew, even after everyone has had second or third bowls. Do we compost the food, or put it in containers that will become trash? I struggle similarly with leftovers at restaurants.

In an ideal world, people will have homes to cook in, and will carry reusable containers with them to transport any leftover food so they can eat it later (always getting it into a fridge within two hours, as per good food safe practices). Until we get there, we need creative ways of both thinking through the chaos of living on the margins, and the high-waste lifestyle we have adopted.

The conversation with city staff encouraged me. It felt good to have a role at a significant table, and to have something to contribute. I recognize the privilege of getting to move between food lines and city officials. I had been feeling a little rundown, dispirited by a mediocre class I facilitated earlier in the week, and by several conversations I had with colleagues who are focusing on aspects of our support systems that I do not see as relevant. That meeting helped me see how the different threads to which I am drawn all weave together. I was reminded of what strands we need to make our tapestry of care more beautiful, and less likely to allow people like Mak, Neil, and Meg to slip through.

Chapter 8

Another Way of Being

Trusting the Spirit to Lead

Whenever I hear the "May the road rise up to meet you" prayer, I remember one of my first meals at the Oasis Café, when it was still using a busy food line format. The person I was replacing was orienting me to the people and rhythms of the program, but the only detail that remains with me is that Ron, one of the guests, was particularly belligerent that day. You learn the names of the agitators first. Ron would not leave when asked, so Carmen, who was orienting me to the coordinator role, told him she was going to call the police. He did leave when he realized she was seriously dialing the authorities, and did not cause issues again, though for a long time I felt a heightened awareness whenever he came for a meal. Thankfully, there were only a few people like this. The majority are gracious guests.

At that time, it had been the tradition, just before lunch was served, for the program coordinator to welcome everyone, share any announcements, and ask if one of the dinner guests would give thanks for the meal. I often wished I had recorded the earnestly beautiful prayers. One day, after I had finished my welcome speech and invited someone to pray, the only person who stood up was

Ron. I scanned the other side of the room, willing someone else to offer, but when no one did, I made eye contact with Ron, giving him permission (reluctantly) to say the grace. I have learned to trust the Spirit to lead in these moments, though it is a lesson I will have to learn over and over.

Ron bowed his head and said in a loud, raspy voice, "May the road rise up to meet us, may the wind be at our backs, and may there always be a hell of a lot of women here."

Then he sat down.

In the silence that followed, I knew the rest of the hungry guests were looking at me for direction, or obediently keeping their eyes closed until I indicated that the prayer was over. I internally debated whether I should say "amen" and honor his prayer, or use this as a moment to model what we mean when we offer grace before a meal. Fortunately, another guest stood up and thanked God for the food, and for all the people who made the meal possible. At that point it felt right to say "amen" and invite the first table up to get their food.

In 2009, I started a Masters in Healthcare Leadership. I had been looking to do some further studies, but did not want to do clinical research. What I needed to know about nutrition I learned on the job, reading up on specific topics as they presented themselves, and so I looked for a multidisciplinary program with which to engage. If I am to be honest, I mostly wanted to avoid a thesis, although looking back, writing my thesis, which ended up being called "A Journey that Takes Time" (though its working title was "Derailed by Bacon," as it almost was), was one of the highlights of the degree. "You will be underwhelmed by the simplicity of your research, and overwhelmed by what you can pull out of it," a professor had told me when I was starting the process. It was true.

Ultimately, the deciding factor in my choice of that program—aside from my dad encouraging me, the school being in Victoria where I had some loved ones, and my frustration at my inability to address the complex systemic challenges hindering my colleagues and I from implementing a new approach to hospital food in Greater Vancouver (though I was halfway through my degree before I could articulate that)—was a comment made by a recent graduate I had connected with. He said that the program teaches you to think differently. Many are talking and writing about leadership eloquently, so I will add just the three most poignant things I have learned, or what is most relevant as I learn to engage with my hungrier neighbors.

Leadership as a Way of Being

First, leadership is a way of being, not necessarily a position. I do not remember who first articulated this idea to me, but it allowed me to start identifying with leadership roles, and then sharing them with those who have little experience leading others.

"Karen, Karen!" Lou rushed over to me a few minutes before opening doors to the guests at a community meal. The urgency in her voice made me wonder if there was a fire in the building, or we were out of sugar, or if there was some other reason serious enough to cancel the night's meal. There were a lot of details to pull together, but I stopped what I was doing and gave her my full attention, bracing myself to sort out the crisis. I held the leadership role in this program, but I was trying to share that with the people who came as guests, many of whom had few opportunities for ownership, and even fewer experiences with healthy power dynamics.

"It was my birthday and my daughter made me roast beef! And potatoes with melted cheese on them," Lou told me proudly, with emphasis on the *melted cheese*. Maybe she was hinting that we should serve cheesy potatoes one day. Maybe she thought the gourmet touch would impress me. Probably, she has a deep well inside that is open to affirmation, and has lived through some chaotic, hungry years. Now that her life is settling, though her apartment had suffered severe smoke damage a few weeks before this conversation, she was secure enough with her role in this group that she could ask for validation in her indirect way. I have learned enough to make space to give it, even if it means dinner will be a few minutes late. When Lou opened the doors to our guests, she did so confidently, if a bit bossily on occasion, keeping closer tabs than I could on who had come and how sober they were.

Living Systems

Secondly, leadership school taught me to see living systems. As we learned new terms and frameworks for the complex, dynamic networks in which we exist, I became increasingly intrigued. No moment is just a moment.

We tend to see our programs and organizations as machines—if we adjust one factor, or put in a certain fuel, we expect a particular outcome. But people, especially the colorful ones who tend to show up in community food programs, constitute more of an ecosystem, where we can hope for, but not guarantee, certain reactions. Our dinner guests, like people around the world, each come with their unique needs and history. Even when staying in a center that provides ample structure and fuel (food), we will still encounter surprising responses that can throw the whole ecosystem out of balance.

I arrived at a center one day to a string of messages from the security and support staff, who were trying to figure out how to address a client who had been caught carrying "2 sandwiches, 1 bottle of juice, 4 individual cupcakes, and a package of 12 cupcakes under his hoodie up to his room. He said he was allowed because he is diabetic."

Although it was an impressive feat if he had carried all that from the nearest corner store, which was at least a few blocks away, the client presented a problem for several reasons. No food was allowed in rooms, as former tenants had not proven themselves to be competent housekeepers and their crumbs had attracted small critters. Hiding anything under one's clothing, or any such secretive behavior, disregards the honesty and self-revelation that must be the basis for any recovery program. And sixteen cupcakes? No one needs that many, even if his body's ability to control blood sugar was stellar. It took a number of us who were part of that client's network to address the sixteen-cupcake level transgression.

Just as we constantly regenerate cells, yet can still be recognized, our ecosystems evolve, yet a recognizable stability remains. Our programs need to learn this generative cycle from the natural world. I have worked with several organizations that run two or more meal programs a week, each led by a different volunteer team, and thus each developing its own culture and way of doing things. It is confusing to the guests to come into the same space but be expected to get their food in different ways. People are to wait to be served coffee or have their dishes collected some days, and supposed to do it themselves other days, maybe even getting reprimanded by a well-meaning volunteer because they did not understand the system *du jour*. We cannot overestimate how much people with otherwise chaotic lives appreciate consistency. While renewing and refining our way of doing things is good, it is valuable to have someone who holds institutional memory, and who watches out for those who need a little more facilitating into a new way of being.

Knowledge + Solution

The third significant leadership idea I learned is that, while we say knowledge is power, it is articulating knowledge + a solution that leads to good action. I had coffee recently with someone who is in my gray zone of friend-volunteer-program participant. I wanted to know her opinion on what makes for a good meal, as I was part of a team planning for a new community meal in a part of Vancouver were three other food programs had shut down in the past few years. While I do not know much about the decision-making process of the churches and organizations that ran these meals, it appears that they shut down, at least in part, because leadership was not shared with guests, and the original volunteer team ran out of steam.

As we chatted over lattes, my friend told me about a group that had wanted to use a common space in her social housing unit for a social enterprise, but she and her neighbors had resisted. They had succeeded in stopping the plan, as they had not liked how the idea had been presented. The group, which was doing some great work, was now struggling to find a new space. Then she told a few stories of other things she had blocked or opposed. I left the meeting with a few good ideas, but mostly tired out.

As I walked back home, I thought about why our conversation had felt so draining, and then about comments one of my professors had made. It is not wrong to oppose things, but to simply complain makes no one's job easier. There are times to lead up, when it can be effective to tell those in charge of any system about problems experienced at your level, but this is best accompanied with an idea to change the problem. Those in leadership may see the larger system and have a valid reason for why one action may or may not be viable, but they often can work with suggestions for addressing issues.

Connect Before You Correct

Another core part of *leadership as a way of being* relates to wise and ethical decision-making. As with strength training, we develop the ability to make the right decision in any complex moment by exercising our little ethical muscles so they are brawny and beefy when they need to make a bigger moral choice. We need to see those in leadership make smaller principled decisions, so we trust them enough to bring larger, trickier issues to them for consultation.

One night, in the middle of a community meal, Erica, a guest, somehow thought Mike, another guest, looked at her maliciously. Unnerved, she asked him to stop. Knowing Erica, I can imagine that she asked this rather unkindly, to which Mike replied, "Your tone of voice offends me, and I would like to be treated with more dignity," or something like that. I was not in the room during this exchange, so I will make an educated guess that those were not the words he used, but they do reflect his feelings. At least his deeper feelings. If he were not so agitated, he might have articulated that he was hurt, and shifted what happened next.

I walked into the dining room as the argument was heating up. Without really thinking, I planted myself between the two, and simultaneously tried to get Erica to leave the building and Mike to calm down. This was complicated by Erica screaming, "He's harassing me!" Such a plea must always be taken seriously, though, as with the boy-who-cried-wolf, it was hard to see Erica as an innocent victim when she claims she is harassed almost every visit, and is usually the only one to make such claims.

The moment was also complicated when two male volunteers, either wanting to protect me, or who were just triggered by the rising tensions, raced up and started yelling at Mike, further agitating him. We somehow got the two vocal volunteers and Erica out of the room, making it clear to Erica that she should leave the property. I then sat down at the table with Mike as he finished his meal. We talked about what happened, and he got upset, then calm, upset, then calm, several times. Thankfully, Carlos, a volunteer gifted with reserve and understanding, sat down with us. He seemed to slip into an easy conversation with Mike, and I excused myself to check on everything else.

As I stood up, I was asked by a new volunteer if he could sit in on the Bible study hosted for the meal guests. I walked him down the hall toward the room where the group was gathered, explaining that it would likely feel a little different from other discussions he had been part of, given the mix of eccentric believers and hostile agitators that made up the core of the group. As I quietly ushered him into the room, I saw Erica in the circle. I later learned that she had gone around the outside of the church building and knocked on the window where the group was meeting, signaling that she wanted to be let in.

Was this an act of defiance, and should that result in barring Erica for a few weeks? It was not fair to allow inappropriate behavior without consequences. Or was her joining the Bible study an honest seeking of community and grace, and thus should I encourage it? Or at least permit it, and forget her earlier outburst? I was pretty sure she joined the group out of rebelliousness, not humility, but decided to give Erica the benefit of the doubt and let her stay.

While I wrestled with what to do about Erica, Patrick, another guest, asked me to help him leave and avoid Mike, who was now in the back alley. It seemed wise to help avoid another encounter with Mike, especially as it was almost 8:30 pm, and we try to not annoy our neighbors. I walked Patrick through an exit on the south side of the building and then accompanied him a block up the street in the direction of the shelter he was staying that night. As I turned back toward the church, I heard Mike yelling again.

This time, Mike was ruffled by a small, yappy dog, that seemed to be equally triggered by Mike. I ran down the block and did my best to divert Mike's attention until the dog and its owner were far enough away. Again, Mike cycled rapidly through anger, calm, anger, and calm. He did not know why people were too stupid to train their dogs. He apologized to me for the outburst. He was still mad at Erica. He thanked me for the meal. He did not know where he was going that night and that upset him. He appreciated my kindness. He was pissed at the person who stole his bag. He was proud to show me his bike.

At one point, when he started to get agitated again, I asked if I could pray. I cannot explain how I knew it was safe to stand in that dark alley with him, or stand between him and Erica earlier in the evening, or that it was the right time to pray. These things are only learned by experience. Mike seemed to be taken off guard by my question. From comments he had made earlier, I had gathered that he had some Faith, but his experience with church had not been entirely positive.

"Oh. Yeah. Okay. Sure. So, Jesus is your mascot?" was his response.

"Yeah, something like that," I said, smiling with him. And then, with the tension slipping away, I expressed thankfulness for meeting Mike that night. It did not feel right to pray for anything more. It was amazing how Mike's demeanor changed in those few minutes.

Mike left, but I still wrestled with how to address Erica. By allowing her to stay, I was making peace for the short term, but maybe creating problems for the next time she visited. I was showing grace to her, but not fairness to the larger community. If she were forced to leave, would she go to another program or café and cause trouble? Likely. If her behavior had no consequences, would she grasp that it is wrong to stir up controversy or ignore me when I asked her to leave for the night? Probably not.

Connect before you correct, is what my wise friend Karen would say. Erica certainly would not hear any well-thought out arguments from me if I pulled her out of the study group. I decided it was not the time to address anything with her. We could talk next time we shared a meal together.

Right-Versus-Right Decisions

In a course on ethics, I learned to consider the right-versus-right decisions we have to make as constituting a choice; for example, between an individual or a group, or between short- and long-term consequences, or justice versus mercy. In most situations, best choices will have some negative consequences, too.

Another day, I found myself in my office, sitting with Tim, who was clean-cut, articulate, and not at all the person I expected, given what I had heard about him. Tim was just out of jail, having served nine years for criminally crossing another person's boundaries. In the few weeks he had been at the center, he had earned himself a reputation for being manipulative, entitled, and difficult to feed. I had been asked to meet with him to help address the latter issue, and warned about his way of relating.

After asking my standard questions on medical history and appetite, I asked Tim about his vegetarianism, and whether he had decided to avoid meat for health, ethics, or preference. Whether in a clinical setting or at a dinner party, this question usually leads to interesting conversation.

"Ethics, I guess," was his response. "When I was inside, I got to thinking about how I could make things right with my life, and the only thing I could think of was to stop eating animals. It is bad how they are raised. I doubt they give us good meat in jail. I tried going vegan, but that was too hard."

We talked about protein options available to him, why the cooks at the center could not always make what he was asking for, given the hundreds of other meals they were making each day, and what a healthy vegetarian diet looked like.

We discussed the idea of being *flexitarian*—generally eating in a way that fits your chosen values, but occasionally eating other food when what you want is not available. Tim considered this for a moment, then explained that he had an extreme personality, and needed to be all in or all out. Only once, when he had been given a burger in jail, had he eaten meat in the past few years. He was told it was vegetarian, and had wondered how it could taste so meaty. When he inquired, the server realized his mistake, and told Tim the burger had actually been beef. Tim told me he had not been upset. Everyone makes mistakes. I wondered, though not out loud, how that scene had really played out.

I spent the rest of the afternoon working on a guide for the cooks at that center on making vegetarian and vegan meals. It was a project I had been meaning to work on for a few months, and finally made the time to complete it. I knew I had to consider the budget, space, and time constraints of the facility, but as we think about our food choices, we have to acknowledge the abyss between what we do to animals, and what we ought to practice in light of all we know. The guide primarily focused on the nutritional appropriateness and practicality of the food served to clients who choose to not eat animals, but it was another nudge for the facility into a better practice. By addressing the callous ways animals are treated in our food systems, we can also end some of the inhumane working conditions created in our quest for cheap meat. Vulnerable people get stuck with the worst jobs on factory farms and processing plants. Eating fewer animals, and choosing more ethically-raised animals when we do consume them, will also address some pressing environmental challenges, health concerns, excessive antibiotic use, and overall food insecurity.

We are starting to use terms like *social procurement*, or making purchasing choices that are not just transactional (exchanging money for goods), but have transformative potential for our community, by adding to human capital (individuals gaining skills and connections), cultural capital (fostering diversity and respect), and physical capital (positively impacting the natural world). Adding in such considerations when deciding what to purchase for a community program quickly gets complex, but hopefully we will get to the point where we look back on this era and wonder how we could have let our food systems get to the state they are in, or let anyone live without a basic income equivalent to a living wage that allows them to participate in constructive social procurement.

While I worked on the guide, I mulled over the conversation I had with Tim, and others before him. He was not my first client who was exploring ethical eating as part of his journey toward recovery and reintegration. Was it an act of justice, in this instance, to make Tim eat what was being served to everyone else, or was it more important to show mercy, and make special food for him? Was it appropriate to ask the cooks, servers, and dishwashers to do extra work to prioritize this individual's request? Would extra accommodations make a difference when Tim left the center and began the next season of life? How important is it to honor a commitment like vegetarianism, helping someone make amends for past mistakes?

My mind wrestled for the rest of the afternoon, being a bit too hard on myself for the lack of compassion that I felt for Tim, or the temptation (that I would barely admit to myself) to further punish him by not giving him the privilege of good meatless entrées. At one point, I happened to be walking past a recycling bin when another client, obviously new to the program and still very fatigued, shuffled toward me in faded pajamas. He had just finished a juice box when he made vague eye contact with me and asked if he could recycle his container in the blue box. I told him he could, hope restored that someone in his state still cared about reducing waste.

"Thanks," he said. Then he added, "You are doing a good job," as he shuffled on down the hall.

Stealing Vegetables

Another day, when I was leading a group discussion in a supportive program, the conversation settled on extreme behaviors. Someone shared that, when he eats or drinks, even water or healthy foods, he cannot stop himself, and consumes an excessive amount. Unsurprisingly, a few others admitted similar tendencies. At points like this, I sometimes ask the group if they remember the term *homeostasis* from high school science class. I explain, as simply as I can, about our body's hormones and mechanisms which maintain its preferred internal temperatures and blood sugar levels, and if we let ourselves get into an extreme state—be it hungry, thirsty, fatigued, over-stimulated, cold, or hot—our instincts take over and we feel a strong drive to do whatever it takes to get back in balance. The need for basic self care and the impact of pushing our bodies too far usually seems to make sense to individuals in early stages of recovery.

One guy in this group still needed to get something off his chest. "I crave salads sometimes," he explained. I nodded, encouraging him to go on, hopeful that this would turn into a story about how he feels better when he consumes leafy green vegetables. This was not the setting to explain our bodies' need for folate and non-heme iron, but I could encourage salad eating, especially now that a salad bar was set up at every lunch and dinner at the facility.

The guy continued, "I go to the store, and get one of those salads in a box, well, I steal it, but when I get them, I want to eat the whole thing." I knew that the group had a short attention span, and I only had a few more minutes with them. I had to choose between mentioning the salad bar and addressing his admission of stealing food.

A few minutes before, we had been talking about what microwaves do to food. There is often someone in this type of setting who harbors conspiracy theories about what microwaves, or preservatives, or other modern inventions do to us. Someone had commented that we could not get away from things like that, "because almost everything we eat is microwaved now." I also wanted to go back and explore that statement. It was probably true that much of what the people in the room had consumed in the months leading up to their stay in the program had been ultra-processed and microwaved, and although the reasons for addiction are deep and complex, a poor diet contributes to one's inability to make good decisions.

Sensing that it was time to wrap up the discussion, I ended with the idea that it takes time for our body rhythms to return to normal, and there was no quick fix for health. The individuals in the group would find a good cadence of digestion, elimination, sleep, energy, and moods as they moved through the recovery process. I had to trust that everyone knew that stealing vegetables was not an approach I endorsed.

Telling the Truth About Bavarian Smokies

In the ethics course mentioned above, we talked about priorities in situations where there is more than one right response. Another lens through which to view this challenge is to recognize that some people are truth-seekers, while others are peace-seekers. I tend to be the latter. There are times when I can hold truth somewhat lightly, if it means I can love someone a little more lavishly.

One night, at a community dinner, William caught my attention as I walked by him. William is one of Vancouver's more colorful homeless men, both literally and figuratively. That night he was wearing a vibrant purple cowboy hat, which looked like it had been through a few rodeos, though William told me he had bought it the week before with his Goods and Services Tax rebate. He seemed to assume that I agreed he had made a worthy investment with the extra little treat the government gave him.

A year or two earlier, I had been driving a friend to the airport. It was a warm, summer morning, so we had the windows rolled down. We were stopped at a red light, and I looked over and saw William on the sidewalk across the street, holding a large bouquet of flowers, which I am quite sure were pilfered from local gardens. He recognized me, jumped up, ran across the street, and thrust his flowers into my window, saying something like, "Karen, such an absolute pleasure to see you this fine day." Just then, the light turned green and traffic started to move. I thanked William, and before I could say anything else, he ran back across the street.

"Does this kind of thing happen to you often?" my friend asked. I do receive flowers rather frequently, which I appreciate, though I do not endorse stealing, and any hopeful suitors need to understand that I do not consider eating together at a community dinner as a first date.

After William finished telling me about his new hat, he told me, just as earnestly, that he had not received any meat when his meal was brought to him. The plate in front of him contained the salad and roast potatoes we had made that evening, and what looked like a very sausage-shaped line of sauce. I am just shy of one hundred percent certain that our volunteer team would not have forgotten to put a sausage on his plate, and that the person serving as his waiter would not have eaten or traded away the sausage in the few steps from our servery to William's table.

My initial inclinations were to say, "Do you really think I'm that naïve?" or, "How would you feel if you came later, and there was no food left because other people had claimed more than their share?" But I have decided to err on the side of generosity whenever I can, so I brought him another plate. Whether or not William was consciously trying to manipulate me, I am sure he was craving protein and validation. Responding to his needs openhandedly would nourish him more than truth-seeking in the moment.

I got a quiet scolding later from the eagle-eyed volunteer maître d' who had observed my interaction with William. From her vantage point, I had let myself be clearly duped, but she accepted my authority and my explanation. There may have been other right responses to the mysteriously missing sausage, and to similar instances where our vulnerable neighbors lack what they need, but when we believe in abundance, we can make decisions like that.

Conclusion

I WISH I COULD say this is a story of accomplishment. I wish I could say that the food line where I handed out 437 trays without dropping one has transitioned to a more dignified setting, and is on its way to being made redundant. I wish I could say that all of my vulnerable friends have a secure home, a stocked kitchen, and someone to cook with. I wish I could say that the food I order for community programs, and my own grocery list, primarily has items that were ethically sourced. I wish I could say I am more consistently acting like Jesus, even remembering to *consider the lilies*, as He poetically suggested, reminding us to not worry, and to be conscious of how our lives connect with the natural world. I wish my colleagues and I knew how to hold the tension between focusing on immediate needs for food and longer-term, systemic shifts toward a sustainable food system. But this story is part of a larger journey, and we still have work to do.

It took me several years to write down these stories, and even longer to learn their significance within the tapestry of care that is spread across Vancouver. Good things are happening, yet it feels like our tapestry is unraveling in some corners, even as we continue to weave it. Neil has lived in a small apartment for most of the past year, and his skin is notably better, but both Marcus and Brady passed away recently. I can only pray they were not alone in the end, hungry and in pain. I will never know what became of their lives after our last shared meal, but I do take comfort in believing that Marcus no longer needs his arm sling, and Brady now has access to an endless supply of heavenly underwear.

Despite the grief that is so woven into this world, and the *hunger amidst plenty*, this is, in some ways, an unfolding story of accomplishment. We may not get the recipe exactly right, but there are some indicators that we are on track. If our community dinner participants, volunteers, and our guests-become-hosts return week after week—which they will if you love them—we can be encouraged that we are doing something right. And by *love*, I mean providing some good base ingredients and then putting people to work together. If you are looking for something to measure, there are two (almost quantifiable) indicators of success.

First, if your compost bucket is full by the time your meal is ready, that is generally a good sign. Any meal that includes freshly prepared vegetables is going to be good for you. If you check to see if the compost bin is even fuller after the meal, that is called a *plate-waste audit*. I trust it is obvious to rate how well that particular meal had been received.

And second, we know that we are nourishing our vulnerable neighbors, and ourselves, when we regularly experience a sense of awe. We are in the right place when we recognize the abundance around us and feel amazement as we witness the indomitable human spirit. Through breaking bread, or sharing food, we learn what some of *the least of these brothers and sisters* of ours endure, and this inspires compassion, not judgment.

I acknowledge that it is often my own internal barometer that dictates whether I see beauty or harshness in the individuals I meet, and that indicates how hopeful I am that it is worth going to work day after day, doing little things that might help others to experience that feeling of awe. When I am disciplined enough to maintain the rhythms I talk about with my clients—listening to my hunger and satiety cues, balancing what feeds my body, mind, heart, and spirit, and hydrating enough—I experience that sense of awe again and again. Sometimes I have to carve out the time to see it, bribing myself with water that was boiled and steeped in tea leaves, but as I savor my steaming cup, I can usually recognize the significance of the interesting, hard, funny, poignant interactions I witnessed and experienced that day. Often, I need to connect with the people you met on these pages to regain a good perspective.

The head chefs of the larger charities in Vancouver will gather soon, swapping stories, questions, and particularly abundant donations. We affectionately call our group the *Excess Bread Support Group*. Some new faces will be welcomed to the circle, and we will figure out which of our colleagues need a little extra support in this season. We will spend some time imagining how we can nourish, a little more creatively, those who are struggling the most in Vancouver. I feel awe and appreciation when I am amongst this group, as I am reminded that I can tap into a wealth of experience when I need it.

Meals will be served and dishes washed in homes and church halls across this city. I have a pot of black beans cooking as I write this, preparing for my extended family who will gather this weekend for dinner, and for my household, at least some semblance of us, who will gather this evening around our table. When I am amongst these circles, I feel that same awe, and that same appreciation for the warmth and familiarity of our regular connections. When food shifts from being a chore to a sacrament, something human wakes up in us.

One of the servers at a neighborhood program writes clever bits of recovery wisdom on the paper chef's hat he puts on everyday. I took a photo of this one, and pull it up whenever I feel daunted by the project stretching out before me. Whether it is the recovery journey, or just a big dinner party, there is some truth in this if we look for it:

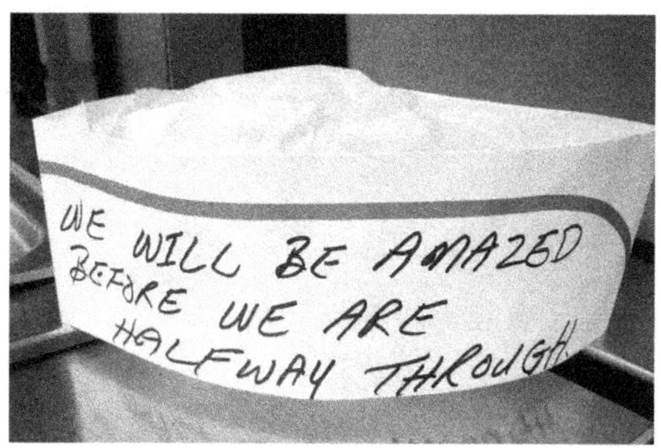

The title *Happy Colon, Happy Soul* started as a joke, descending into a bit of *potty humor* that should cease to be funny after we reach double digits, but as with all good humor, it illustrates something significant. What we eat influences our gut health, which influences our emotional health, and thus all the interactions we experience and decisions we make throughout the day. *Gut feelings* always point to something legitimate, and probably have our best interests at heart.

As you plan your next meal, whether it is for yourself, or for a few hundred hungry neighbors, consider how we are sated with beauty and astonishment, and that, like the food we eat, we need to feast on these regularly. I recently sat down to eat near the end of a community dinner with a volunteer who had become part of the program's core team. We had made it through the hour of chaos where we wonder if the meal will ever come together (though is always does), and had found two chairs in a corner of the hall. There was a moment of silence between us as we took the first few bites of our food and watched our guests chatting over their dinners, with evergreen branches on the tables and soft string lights brightening up the space. "I love this," she said, grasping what can only be experienced. Like food, reading about it is not as satisfying as living it.

There are so many awe-inspiring moments emanating from the beauty, the messiness, the complexity, and the joy of shared meals. I hope these stories have helped you fall in love with my extended family, or at least to see Vancouver, or your city, a little differently.

Bibliography

Boyle, Greg. *Tattoos on the Heart* (United States: Simon and Schuster, 2011).

Brooks, David. *The Road to Character* (New York: Random House, 2016).

Brown, Brené. *Rising Strong: How the Ability to Reset Transforms the Way We Live, Love, Parent, and Lead* (London: Vermilion, 2015).

Escobar, Kathy. *Down We Go: Living into the Wild Ways of Jesus* (Folsom, CA: Civitas Press, 2011).

Ladner, Peter. *The Urban Revolution: Changing the Way We Feed Cities* (Gabriola Island: New Society Publications, 2012).

Miles, Sara. *Take This Bread: a Radical Conversion* (London: Canterbury Press Norwich, 2012).

Oliver, Mary. *Red Bird* (Tarset: Bloodaxe, 2008).

Pious Society of St. Paul. *Blessed Mother Teresa* (London: St Pauls, 2003).

Pollan, Michael. *Food Rules: An Eater's Manual* (Camberwell, Vic: Penguin, 2010).

Poppendieck, Janet. *Sweet Charity? Emergency Food and the End of Entitlement* (New York: Penguin, 1999).

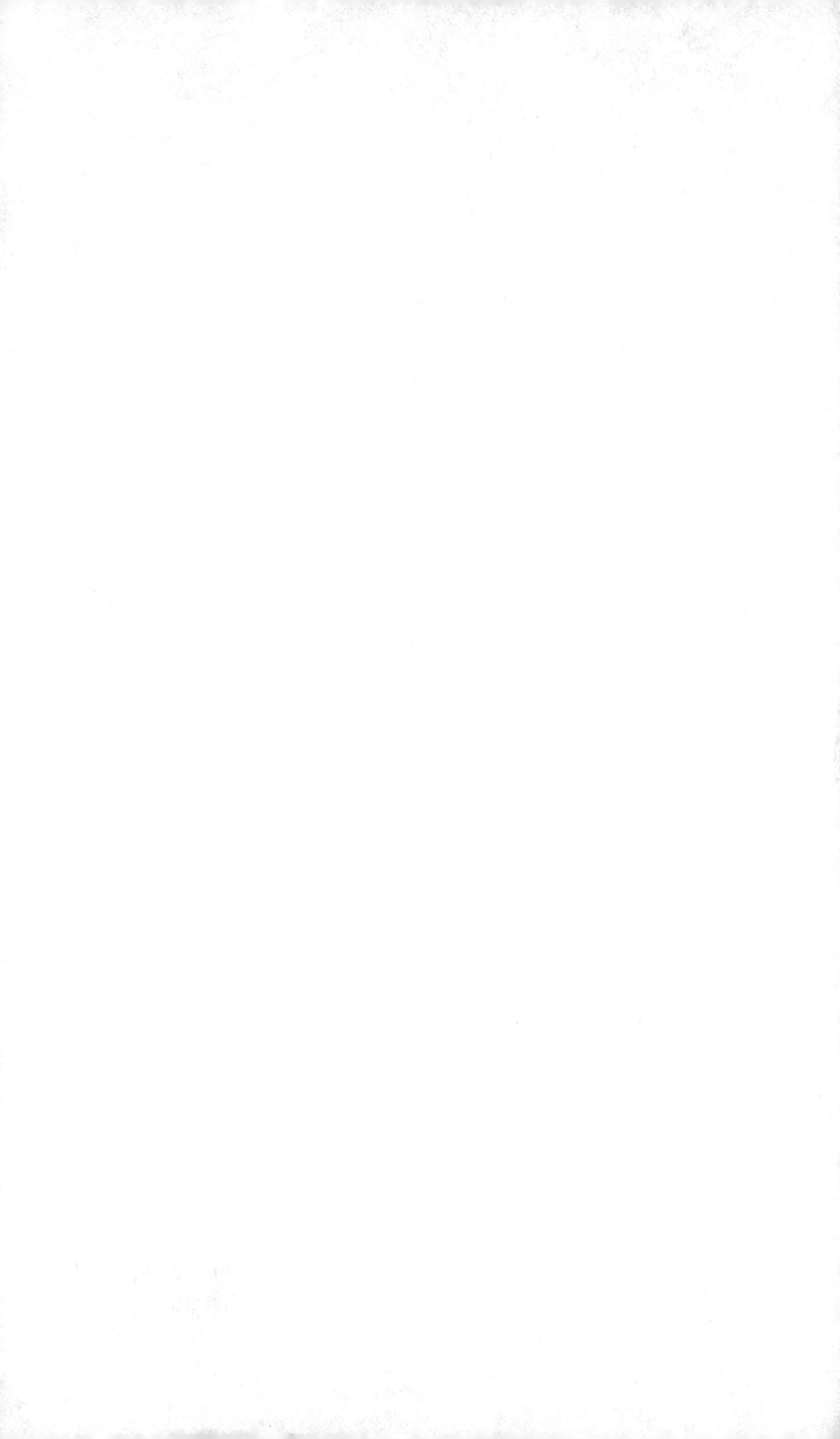

CPSIA information can be obtained
at www.ICGtesting.com
Printed in the USA
LVHW080143110719
623746LV00001B/1/P

9 781532 682254